Current issu
hypertension

Current issues in hypertension

Neil R Poulter MB, Msc, FRCP

Professor of Preventive Cardiovascular Medicine,
Imperial College, London, UK

Always refer to the manufacturer's Prescribing Information before prescribing drugs cited in this book.

British Library Cataloguing in Publication Data

A catalogue record for this title is available from the British Library

ISBN 1-904218-30-X

Neil R Poulter

Current issues in hypertension

Design and production:

Design Online Limited, 21 Cave Street, Oxford OX4 1BA

Printed by

Halstan & Co Ltd, Amersham, Bucks HP6 6HJ, UK

Distributed by

Plymbridge Distributors Ltd, Estover Road, Plymouth PL6 7PY, UK

Contents

Introduction — vii

1 Epidemiology — 1
Definition of hypertension — 2
Distribution of hypertension — 5
Aetiology of raised BP — 9
Natural history of hypertension — 13

2 How should patients with hypertension be assessed? — 25
BP measurement — 26
Medical History — 29
Examination — 30
Investigations — 30
Global risk assessment — 31

3 At what level should drug treatment be initiated? — 43
Patients at < 20% risk of a major cardiovascular event in the next 10 years — 44
Patients with established vascular disease or at high risk of developing it (> 20% 10-year cardiovascular risk) — 44

4 Is non-drug treatment worthwhile? — 53
Evidence — 54
Non-drug measures and antihypertensive medication — 56

5 How far should BPs be lowered? — 59

6 What drug treatment should be used — 65
Trial evidence as of 1993/94 — 66
Benefits of more contemporary drugs over standard therapy — 67
What is the optimal pair of BP-lowering agents? — 78
Which drugs are best for different sub-groups of patients? — 83

7 What concomitant therapy is needed? **95**

Which patients with hypertension merit lipid-lowering therapy? 96

ALLHAT-LLT and ASCOT-LLA studies 97

Which patients with hypertension should receive aspirin? 98

Which patients with hypertension should receive antioxidant
therapy? 98

8 How to improve BP control **101**

How well is BP treated and controlled? 102

Why is hypertension managed so inadequately? 102

Can we improve BP control? 105

9 What are the prospects for the future? **109**

What don't we know? 110

How to improve implementation of guidelines 111

Will more effective modification become available? 113

Population vs high-risk strategy 115

Index **119**

Introduction

Hypertension has more data available from major randomised trials to guide practice, than almost any other area of medicine.

Despite this extensive and ever-expanding database, there are still several major unanswered questions regarding the optimal management of hypertension. This book attempts to outline the data relating to these issues, and provides a résumé and critique of how contemporary recommendations in recent sets of national and international guidelines deal with these areas of uncertainty.

The first chapter briefly outlines the epidemiology of blood pressure (BP) because the distribution, determinants and natural history of raised BP have a critical impact on the answers to several of the contemporary issues to be discussed. Thereafter, subsequent chapters will raise practical questions relevant to those involved with clinical hypertension management and attempt to provide an update regarding how far the questions have been answered, what current guidance is, and what more needs to be done.

Whilst the data and opinions expressed in this book are likely to be updated and changed in the light of increasing information, it is hoped that, in the meantime, this book might be useful in providing some insight into the difficult unresolved issues surrounding hypertension management and thereby improve the clinical care of patients with raised BP. If this goal is achieved it will represent a small step towards the ultimate goal of reducing the huge global burden of disease due to raised BP, which is expected to increase.

Chapter 1

Epidemiology

Hypertension is currently recognised as one of the major contributors to the global burden of disease.[1] It exerts its adverse impact on cardiovascular events all over the world, whether in developed or developing countries (Fig. 1.1). As one of the most common and easily measurable risk factors for cardiovascular diseases, it affords an excellent starting point for initiating or reinforcing strategies to prevent the intolerable burden of cardiovascular disease to which the world is currently exposed.

Definition of hypertension

Blood pressure (BP) levels are normally distributed in the population.[2] It is also clear, from a prognostic viewpoint, that no distinct subset of the population appears to be abnormal, based on BP level (Fig. 1.2).[3] This has major implications for exactly how hypertension is defined.

In 1969 Pickering said hypertension is 'a disorder hitherto unrecognised in medicine, in which the defect is qualitative and not quantitative. It is difficult for doctors to understand because it is a departure from the ordinary process of binary thought to which they are brought up. Medicine in its present state can count up to two, but not beyond.' Not much has changed in 34 years, in that there is still a tendency to consider hypertension as present or absent.

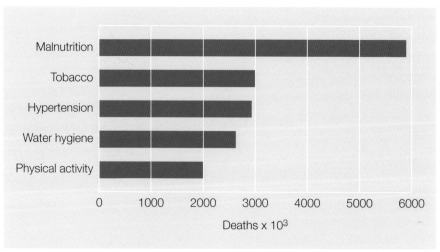

Fig. 1.1 Global disease burden attributable to selected risk factors (1990).

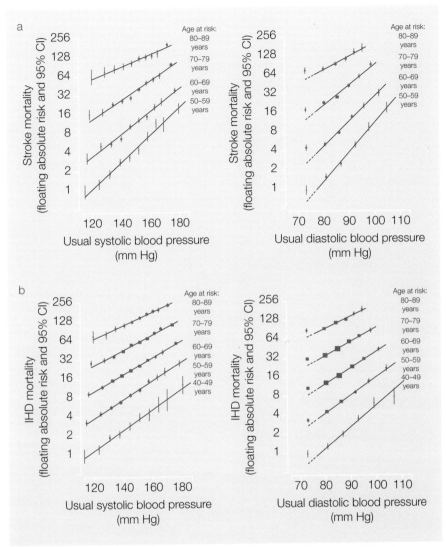

Fig. 1.2 (a) Stroke mortality rate in each decade of age versus usual blood pressure at the start of that decade. Rates are plotted on a floating absolute scale, and each square has area inversely proportional to the effective variance of the log mortality rate. For diastolic BP, each age-specific regression line ignores the left-hand point (i.e. at slightly less than 75 mmHg), for which the risk lies significantly above the fitted regression line (as indicated by the broken line below 75 mmHg). (b) Ischaemic heart disease (IHD) mortality rate in each decade of age versus usual BP at the start of that decade. Conventions as in Figure 1.2a.

However there are several possible ways to classify and define the levels of BP that might be considered as hypertensive, although the decision processes whereby these definitions are determined are to an extent unscientific and arbitrary. The classic method of defining abnormal levels of BP as those outside two standard deviations above the mean is clearly inappropriate since all populations would have a prevalence of hypertension of 5% irrespective of actual BP levels. As shown in Figure 1.2, no obvious level of BP is prognostically associated with the initiation in risk of cardiovascular events, which would allow populations to be dichotomised into normotensive and hypertensive. So, from a pragmatic viewpoint, the working definition of hypertension should be 'that level of BP above which investigation and treatment do more good than harm'.

BP classification	Systolic BP (mmHg)		Diastolic BP (mmHg)
Normal	<120	and	<80
Prehypertension	120–139	or	80–89
Stage 1 hypertension	140–159	or	90–99
Stage 2 hypertension	≥160	or	≥100

Table 1.1a Classification and management of blood pressure for adults (aged ≥18 years).[4]

Category	Systolic	Diastolic
Optimal	<120	<80
Normal	120–129	80–84
High normal	130–139	85–89
Grade 1 hypertension (mild)	140–159	90–99
Grade 2 hypertension (moderate)	160–179	100–109
Grade 2 hypertension (severe)	≥180	≥110
Isolated systolic hypertension	≥140	<90

Table 1.1b Definitions and classification of BP levels (mmHg).[5]

This definition is, by necessity, therefore dependent upon the results of randomised, placebo-controlled clinical trials of the management of raised BP and has implications for BP treatment thresholds, as discussed in Chapter 3, p. 43.

Meanwhile the most recent guidelines[4,5] classify hypertension not so much in terms of randomised, controlled trial (RCT) evidence, but more on the basis of population-based observational data incorporating arbitrary cutpoints for the classifications supplied (Table 1.1, JNC 7 vs ESH/ESH). The term 'prehypertension' for the BP range 120–139 mmHg systolic and 80–89 mmHg diastolic used in the JNC 7 guidelines reflects the fact that BP normally rises with age (see later) but might be criticised for potentially medicalising the majority of the population.

Distribution of hypertension

Age and sex

One legacy from the past, which should be discarded, is that normal and acceptable systolic BP can be calculated by adding the age in years to 100. This approach obviously assumes that it is normal for BP to rise with age. It is true that it is usual for BP to rise with age (Fig. 1.3) but only in populations in which it is usual (or common) to die of coronary heart disease (CHD) or stroke. In westernised societies, systolic BP tends to rise across the whole age range whereas diastolic BP peaks around 60 years in men and later in women, and falls thereafter (Table 1.2).[6]

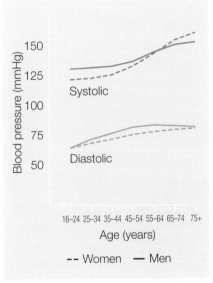

Fig. 1.3 Mean blood pressure levels amongst English adults by age.

Consequently, in those over the age of 65 years, pulse pressure tends to increase and isolated systolic hypertension becomes increasingly common.

	Age (years)								
	16–19	20–29	30–39	40–49	50–59	60–69	70–79	80+	Total
Men, n	303	733	1060	945	822	733	456	170	5222
Systolic BP	126 (0.7)	130 (0.4)	131 (0.4)	133 (0.4)	139 (0.6)	146 (0.7)	150 (1.0)	153 (1.6)	137 (0.2)
Diastolic BP	60 (0.5)	68 (0.4)	73 (0.3)	79 (0.4)	82 (0.4)	82 (0.4)	81 (0.6)	79 (1.0)	76 (0.2)
Women, n	321	882	1259	1118	1023	834	617	253	6307
Systolic BP	120 (0.6)	120 (0.4)	121 (0.3)	127 (0.5)	136 (0.6)	145 (0.7)	156 (0.9)	156 (1.5)	132 (0.3)
Diastolic BP	61 (0.5)	67 (0.5	70 (0.3)	73 (0.3)	75 (0.4)	76 (0.4)	78 (0.5)	77 (0.9)	72 (0.1)

*Values for systolic and diastolic BP are mean (SEM) mmHg.
n = number of subjects.

Table 1.2 Mean systolic and diastolic BP levels by age and gender in 1998 Health Survey of England.[6]

This 'normal' rise of BP with age actually reflects pathological processes in the arterial tree due to chronic exposure to one or more of the major environmental determinants of raised BP.[7] These arterial changes drive the systolic BP even higher and eventually drive the diastolic BP down. It is therefore not surprising that in the elderly, elevated systolic BP is a more important predictor of adverse cardiovascular outcomes than diastolic BP.[3] The truly normal situation, as observed in countries in which CHD and stroke are non-endemic, is one in which BP does not rise with age, once physical maturity has been reached (Fig. 1.4).[8] In these 'low-BP populations' hypertension is either extremely rare or non-existent, consistent with the observation that the rate of rise of BP with age in a population correlates with the prevalence of hypertension.

The prevalence of hypertension is obviously dependent on what definition of hypertension is used. However applying any given standard definition, the prevalence varies dramatically among different populations around the world. In some populations, essential hypertension is completely absent whereas in others, such as some black populations in the USA, the majority of adults are considered to be hypertensive.[9]

A recent large nationally representative survey of adults (aged ≥ 16 years) in England[6] – the Health Survey for England – showed the prevalence of hypertension in England (defined as a systolic BP ≥ 160 mmHg, a diastolic BP ≥ 95 mmHg, or being on treatment for hypertension) to be about 20%, but using a more contemporary definition of ≥ 140 mmHg systolic, ≥ 90 mmHg diastolic or receiving treatment, the prevalence was 42% in men and 33% in women, and the majority of adults over 60 years of age in the UK are 'hypertensive' (Table 1.3).

Systolic and diastolic BP tends to be higher among men than women up to the age of about 70 years, after which women have higher systolic but lower diastolic pressures.[10] BP also shows a geographical gradient, for example being higher in the north than in the south of England, and in the developed world it tends to be higher in lower socio-economic strata, particularly among women.

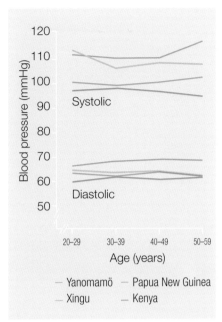

Fig. 1.4 Line graphs of systolic and diastolic pressures by 10-year age groups in four low BP populations.[8]

However the differences in BP that are associated with socio-economic strata appear to be explained largely by higher levels of body mass index in men and women from lower social strata and, among women, by the higher alcohol intakes of those in lower social strata. Finally, BP levels are higher in ethnic minority groups, particularly the African–Caribbean population and, to a lesser extent, the south Asian population.[11]

One recent compilation of data from several national surveys[10] shows that mean BPs in European countries are significantly and consistently higher than in the USA across the age range 35–64 years (Fig. 1.5). It seems unlikely that systematic differences in survey techniques explain these differences and further investigations to explain such findings are in progress. One recent worrisome statistic from surveys in the USA is that hypertension, which had been falling for several decades until 1990, may

	Age (years)								
	16–19	20–29	30–39	40–49	50–59	60–69	70–79	80+	Total
Men, n	303	733	1060	945	822	733	456	170	5222
Percent hypertensive (old definition*)	1.3	1.5	4.0	12.3	25.5	43.4	52.9	54.1	19.8
Percent hypertensive (new definition**)	10.6	20.3	22.6	33.4	52.3	69.4	77.6	81.8	41.5
Isolated systolic hypertension (30+ years), %									
Stage I†	NA	Na	16.0	15.7	26.4	35.9	46.1	49.8	26.6
Stage II‡	NA	NA	0.5	0.4	2.1	8.1	13.8	17.1	4.5
Women, n	321	882	1259	1118	1023	834	617	253	6307
Percent hypertensive (old definition)	0	0.7	2.5	8.5	22.1	41.4	63.5	64.8	20.0
Percent hypertensive (new definition)	3.1	6.1	8.7	21.5	40.8	65.8	82.7	83.8	33.3
Isolated systolic hypertension (30+ years), %									
Stage I†	NA	NA	4.9	13.4	26.0	46.7	57.3	53.1	27.2
Stage II†	NA	NA	0.1	1.2	4.8	13.4	26.1	21.5	8.0

NA indicates isolated systolic hypertension was calculated for those age 30+ years only.
†Systolic BP ≥140 mmHg, diastolic BP <90 mmHg (incorporates stage II).
‡Systolic BP ≥160 mmHg, diastolic BP <90 mmHg
*Systolic BP ≥160 mmHg or diastolic BP ≥95 mmHg or on treatment for hypertension.
**Systolic BP ≥140 mmHg or diastolic BP ≥90 mmHg or on treatment for hypertension.

Table 1.3 Prevalence of hypertension by age and gender in 1998 Health Survey of England.[6]

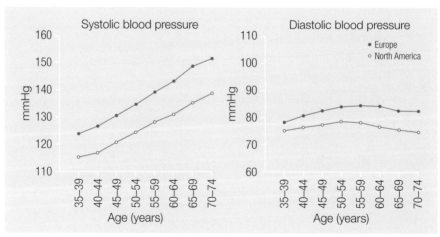

Fig. 1.5 Mean systolic and diastolic BP in six European and two North American countries, men and women combined by age.[10]

have been on the increase between around 1990–2000.[12]

From a worldwide perspective, the prospects for BP levels are daunting. In short, overall BP levels are likely to rise because most of the world is in various stages of development or 'restructuring'. The impact of this process on standard risk factors for BP are shown in Table 1.4. The likely consequences for BP are self-explanatory.

	Rises	Falls
Age	✓	
Exercise		✓
Alcohol intake	✓	
Salt intake	✓	
Potassium intake		✓
Body weight	✓	
Stress	?	
Smoking	✓	
Saturated fats	✓	

Table 1.4 Development and risk factors.

In addition to the impact of development on mean body weight worldwide, an explosion in the prevalence of obesity is occurring throughout the western world (Fig. 1.6).[13] This will inevitably continue to generate an increasing incidence in type 2 diabetes among increasingly younger people.

Diabetes, central obesity and raised BP form three key components of the metabolic syndrome or insulin resistance syndrome.[14] The components of the syndrome are extensive (see Fig. 1.7) and the inter-relationships among these variables is complex. However in the recent National Cholesterol Education Program/Adult Treatment Panel III (NCEP/ATPIII) guidelines[15] the syndrome has been defined on simple clinical grounds as being any three of the five measures shown in Table 1.5, and is considered as a pre-diabetic state.

Aetiology of raised BP

The vast majority of hypertension is described as 'benign' or 'essential'. Given that such hypertension causes a high toll in terms of adverse cardiovascular events and is preventable, these terms are at best unfortunate! However a variable proportion, probably < 10%, are considered as secondary (see Table 1.7). As to the aetiology of essential hypertension, it does appear to be the result of the interaction between

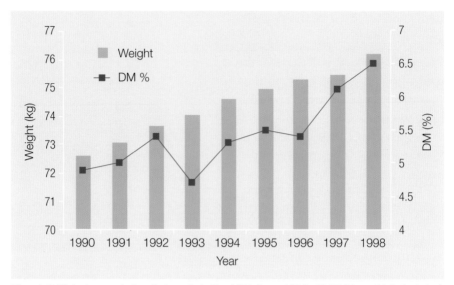

Fig. 1.6 Diabetes and obesity trends in the USA from 1990–1998 (From Mokdad et al. Diab Care 2000; 23: 1278–83).

genetic and environmental influences. The relative impact of these two determinants of the problem is controversial. Nevertheless the vanishingly rare monogenic causes of hypertension (e.g. Liddle's disease) notwithstanding, it seems likely that whatever the genetic component of

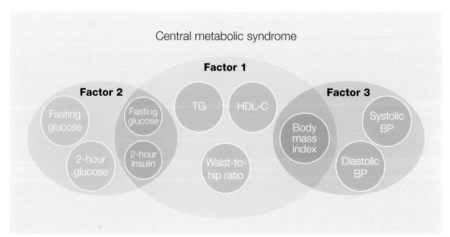

Fig. 1.7 Insulin-resistance syndrome (From Meigs et al. Diabetes 1997; 46: 1594–600).

Metabolic syndrome defined as any 3 of the following variables:

■ Abdominal obesity (waist circumference >102 cm [40 in] in men or >89 cm [>35 in] in women.

■ Glucose intolerance (fasting glucose ≥110mg/dl [≥6.1 mmol/l].

■ BP of at least 130/85 mmHg.

■ High triglycerides (≥150 mg/dl [1.70 mmol/l]).

■ Low high-density liporotein cholesterol (<40mg/dl [<1.04 mmol/l] in men or <50 mg/dl [<1.30 mmol/l] in women.

Table 1.5 Adult Treatment Panel III guideline: Definition of metabolic syndrome.

hypertension, it is polygenic and is less likely to be of value as a target for intervention than the environment – at least for the foreseeable future.

Reference to black African populations undergoing rapid exposure to urbanisation illustrates the potential impact of genes and environmental interactions. Among people living in the UK and USA, higher levels of BP are recognised in those of African descent than in Caucasians.[9,11] However, the prevalence of hypertension is extremely low or non-existent in parts of rural Africa.[8] Migration studies within Africa that tracked those who moved from a rural low-BP setting where hypertension did not exist to an urban environment indicate that the mean BP of the migrating population rises abruptly on arrival in the city.[16] No susceptible subgroup was apparent in terms of elevated BP. In the absence of the environmental change (weight gain, increased sodium intake, decreased potassium intake and raised pulse rates), whatever genetic determinants were at play were not expressed in the remote rural setting.

Identification of some of the genes involved in raised BP may enhance our understanding of the pathogenesis of hypertension and may also serve to characterise those patients who will respond either beneficially or adversely to particular therapies. However, even complete gene mapping is unlikely to lead to a magic therapeutic solution and attention to environmental factors through a population-based approach will remain of prime importance.

Renal artery stenosis	1° Aldosteronism	Corticosteroids
Pylelonephritis	Cushing's syndrome	Liquorice addiction
Obstructive nephropathy	Phaeochromocytoma	Sympathomimetics
Poliomyelitis	Vesico-ureteric reflux	Chromic renal failure
Gout	Porphyria	Adrenal hyperplasia
Diabetes	Acromegaly	Renal JGA tumour
Amyloidosis	Aortic coarction	Glomerulonephritis
Carbenoxalone	↑intracranial pressure	Polycystic kidneys
MAO-inhibitors	Oral contraceptive	Systemic sclerosis
Pre-eclampsia	Endothelinoma	Haemolytic-uremic syndrome
Alcohol	Lead poisoning	

Table 1.6 Some forms or associations of secondary hypertension.

Changes in the nature of our diet from that of our ancestors may hold important clues to the aetiology of hypertension (Table 1.7) and the environmental factors currently considered to be aetiologically associated with raised BP are shown in Table 1.8.

The strength of the evidence supporting the relationship between these variables and hypertension is variably strong. For instance a number of surveys suggest a link between calcium intake and BP, and caffeine intake and BP, but the evidence is inconsistent, even in meta-analyses, and insufficient to recommend modifying dietary calcium or caffeine to either treat or prevent hypertension. Several components of a vegetarian diet (e.g. increased potassium, fibre and vitamin C) may contribute to lower BP and help to explain the lower BPs found among vegetarians. There is good evidence for the involvement of low levels of dietary potassium in raising BP levels and, in addition, low potassium intake is associated with an increased risk of stroke – an association that appears partly independent of BP.[17]

From a pragmatic viewpoint, the evidence relating raised BP with the environment, whilst still controversial for some, is reflected in the non-

Nutrient	Palaeolithic diet (assuming 35% meat)	Current North American diet

Total energy
  protein (%)
  carbohydrate (%)
  fat (%)
	
	30
	45–50
	20–25
		
		12
		46
		42

Polyunsaturated:saturated fat ratio	1.41	0.44
Fibre (g/day)	86	10–20
Sodium (mg)	604	3400
Potassium (mg)	6790	2400
Potassium:sodium ratio	12.1	0.7:1
Calcium (mg)	1520	740

Table 1.7 Estimated diet of late Palaeolithic humans versus that of contemporary North Americans.

pharmacological recommendations for the prevention of the progression of raised BP and the treatment of raised BP, which are included in all recent national and international guidelines (see Ch. 4, p. 54).

Natural history of hypertension

Increasing levels of either an elevated systolic or diastolic BP increase the risk of death (see Table 1.9). Contrary to the emphasis historically placed

- Excess sodium salt intake
- Lack of physical activity
- Overweight
- Insufficient dietary fibre
- Magnesium deficiency
- Excess saturated fats
- Stress
- Alcohol excess
- Low dietary potassium
- Coffee
- Low dietary calcium
- Low vitamin C intake
- Lead exposure

Table 1.8 Environmental determinants of raised BP.

on diastolic pressure after age 50, systolic pressure is a better predictor of subsequent cardiovascular disease than is diastolic pressure (Fig. 1.8).

The macrovascular complications of hypertension are mainly produced by atherosclerotic thrombotic and haemorrhagic vascular disease (Fig. 1.9). Raised BP in humans is associated with a complex pattern of structural changes in the cardiovascular system. These structural changes include:

- Cardiac hypertrophy
- Thickening of the walls of large elastic and muscular arteries
- Remodelling of small muscular arteries, which results in increased wall-to-lumen ratio
- Reduced number of vessels in the microcirculation
- Lengthening of small arteries.

It may be that some aspects of these changes are associated with the initiating process of hypertension, and that others develop as adaptations to the haemodynamic changes – adaptations that may (at least in the first instance) be entirely appropriate.

Systolic BP (mmHg) stratum	Death rate/ 1000	Relative risk	Excess deaths (%)
<110	32.1	1.0	0.0
110–119	34.6	1.1	3.4
120–129	38.0	1.2	12.0
130–139	45.9	1.4	22.5
140–149	55.2	1.7	21.1
150–159	73.2	2.3	18.1
160–169	**82.0**	**2.6**	**9.5**
170–179	**106.1**	**3.3**	**6.1**
≥180	**142.8**	**4.4**	**7.3**

Bold entries are 'high-risk' groups.

Table 1.9 Multiple risk factor intervention trial 'screenees': systolic pressure and age-adjusted all-cause mortality at 10 years. Bold entries are the 'high-risk' group.

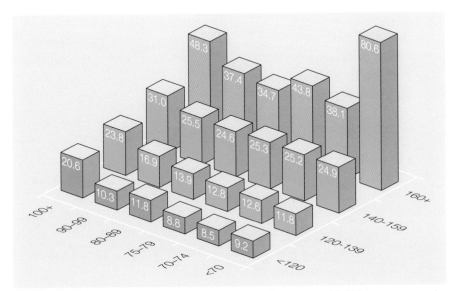

Fig. 1.8 Age-adjusted coronary heart disease death rates per 10,000 person-years by level of SBP and DBP for men screened in the Multiple Risk Factor Intervention Trial. (Reproduced with permission from Neaton JD, Wentworth et al. Cholesterol, blood pressure, cigarette smoking, and death from coronary heart disease. Overall findings and differences by age for 316,099 white men. Arch Intern Med 1992; 152: 56–64).

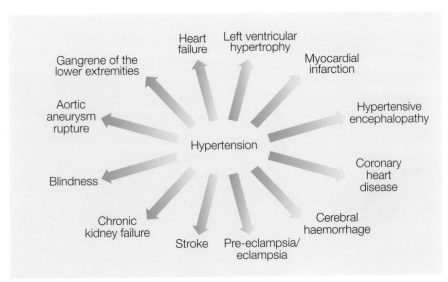

Fig. 1.9 Disease attributable to hypertension.

The vast majority of excess deaths attributable to raised BP are due to CHD, stroke, heart failure, and renal failure. In most parts of the westernised world, the major causes of death currently associated with elevated BP are CHD and stroke, although earlier in the twentieth century renal failure was proportionally more important.

It is important to note that in most of the western industrialised world, although not in other parts of the world, three or four CHD events occur for each stroke event attributable to raised BP (Fig. 1.10). The variable ratios shown in Figure 1.10 reflect the fact that other risk factors interact differentially with raised BP to produce stroke and CHD. This highlights the fact that, although the two disorders share common risk factors, these risk factors are not of equal importance for the two conditions. In short, raised BP is the major risk factor for stroke, whereas abnormal lipids are the key determinant of CHD.

The risk of stroke and CHD events associated with increasing BP levels is shown in Figure 1.2. Importantly because large numbers of people are

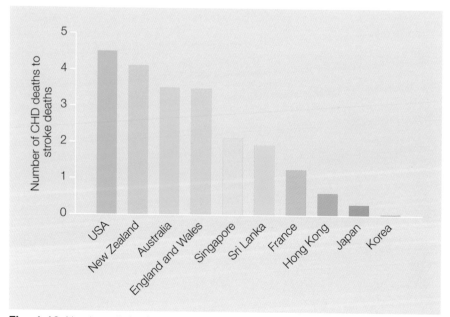

Fig. 1.10 Number of deaths as a result of CHD for each cerebrovascular death in men, 1986–1989.

exposed to a small increase in risk due to slightly raised BP, the majority of strokes and heart attacks attributed to BP occur in people who are conventionally considered 'normotensive' (see Table 1.9). This fact emphasises the importance of the population strategy to lower BP, since focus on those at high risk from raised BP (hypertensives) will not prevent the majority of events due to raised BP.

Hypertension is commonly associated with some degree of renal impairment. In cases of severe essential hypertension, vascular changes within the kidney lead to nephrosclerosis and impairment of renal function. Prior to the introduction of antihypertensive therapy, this resulted in irreversible renal failure. Fortunately, effective antihypertensive treatment now usually prevents the progression of renal disease. Hypertension may, on the other hand, be caused by a primary renal or renovascular pathology, which in some circumstances responds to curative treatment (e.g. angioplasty or surgery for renal artery stenosis).

In patients with hypertension and diabetes, progressive deterioration in renal function is commonly encountered. Good BP control is very important in patients with progressive renal disease of any kind, as emphasised by the drastically diminished survival of haemodialysis patients whose hypertension is inadequately treated.

Although cardiac failure may occur as a consequence of longstanding, untreated hypertension, it is now increasing because of the changing demography of the population and the success of other preventive interventions. Cardiac failure is often preceded by hypertension, but atherosclerotic CHD is probably an equally important contributing factor. The aetiological relationships are therefore complex since hypertension is itself a risk factor for coronary atherosclerosis. Whatever the aetiology, the morbidity and mortality rates associated with heart failure are high (Fig. 1.11).

Hypertension is also the major cause of left ventricular hypertrophy (LVH). The classic cardiac adaptation to sustained hypertension is concentric LVH which consists of left ventricular (LV) wall thickening, as well as an increased LV mass index. However the LV geometry may be normal; the walls may be thick with no increase in LV mass index

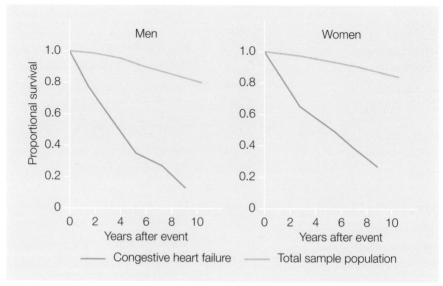

Fig. 1.11 Survival following myocardial infarction: Impact of congestive heart failure.

(concentric remodelling) or the LV cavity may be dilated, which results in an increased LV mass index even though the walls remain a normal size (eccentric hypertrophy) (Fig. 1.12). Compared with normotensive patients, those with hypertension and LVH have a high risk of myocardial infarction and sudden death (Fig. 1.13), which may be related to the increased prevalence of frequent and complex ventricular arrhythmias that have been observed. Both ventricular arrhythmias and sudden death are particularly common in hypertensive patients with LVH as compared with those without.

Obesity and diabetes are also independent causes of LVH and hence, given the frequent coexistence of hypertension with these other two conditions, LVH is commonly found in hypertensive patients. ECG and/or chest radiography are insensitive tests for LVH, but when LVH is detected by either of these methods, there is usually a marked degree of LVH, and therefore it is associated with a significantly worsened cardiovascular prognosis.

At least four observational studies have suggested a link between mid-life or later-life raised BP and subsequent impairment of cognitive

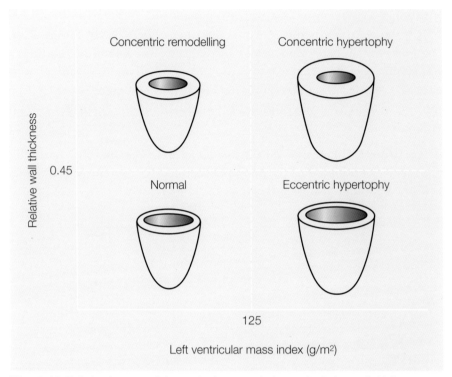

Fig. 1.12 Relation between left ventricular mass index and relative wall thickness

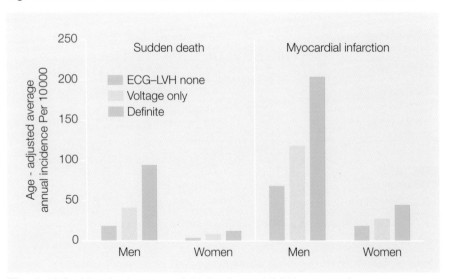

Fig. 1.13 Sudden death, myocardial infarction and LVH in men and women.

function.[18] However to date, data from trials of hypertension treatment have produced conflicting results regarding effects of BP lowering on cognitive function or dementia. Clearly given the ageing of the global population and the fact that the prevalence of dementia doubles with each 5-year rise in age, reaching almost 40% by the ages of 90–95, the possible aetiological role of raised BP in mid-life requires further careful evaluation.

The relative risk of adverse cardiovascular events associated with raised BP appears to be independent of other risk factors. However Table 1.10 shows how the absolute risk of increasing BP is increased by the coexistence

Serum TC (mg/dl)	Systolic pressure (mmHg)					
	<118	118–124	125–131	132–141	142+	Q5/Q1
Non smokers						
<182	3.09	3.72	5.13	5.35	13.66	4.42
182–202	4.39	5.79	8.35	7.66	15.8	3.60
203–220	5.20	6.08	8.56	10.72	17.75	3.41
221–244	6.34	9.37	8.66	12.21	22.69	3.58
245+	12.36	12.68	16.31	20.68	33.40	2.70
Q5/Q1	4.00	3.41	3.18	3.87	2.45	–
Smokers						
<182	10.37	10.69	13.21	13.21	27.04	2.61
182–202	10.03	11.76	19.05	20.67	33.69	3.36
203–220	14.90	16.09	21.07	28.87	42.91	2.88
221–244	19.83	22.69	23.61	31.98	55.50	2.80
245+	25.24	30.50	35.26	41.47	62.11	2.46
Q5/Q1	2.43	2.85	2.67	2.96	2.30	–

Q5 is quintile 5; Q1 is quintile 1. Mean follow-up is 11.6 years.
342,815 men free of heart attack and diabetes at baseline screened for the Multiple Risk Factor Intervention Trial (MRFIT). Excluded from the total of 361,662 men were 8,322 without a baseline SBP reading, 5,440 with a baseline history of MI and 5,625 with a baseline history of diabetes mellitus. Because some men had more than one of these exclusion factors, the total number of men excluded was 18,847.

Table 1.10 Baseline cigarette smoking, quintiles of serum cholesterol, systolic pressure and age-adjusted CHD mortality per 10,000 person-years

of raised cholesterol and smoking. Equally important is the frequent coexistence of some of the major risk factors, particularly hypertension and dyslipidaemia. Dyslipidaemia expressed as total serum cholesterol is more common among hypertensive than normotensive patients, and more commonly involves low levels of high-density lipoprotein (HDL) cholesterol and raised triglycerides as part of the insulin-resistance syndrome.[14]

Figure 1.14 shows the impact on absolute risk of CHD death by increasing quintiles of systolic SBP stratified by quintiles of total serum cholesterol.

Mean lipid levels among hypertensive patients are raised, for example mean total cholesterol (+/– SD) was 6.0 (+/– 1.1) mmol/l (232 mg %) among over 19,000 hypertensive men and women aged 40–79 years who were randomised into a recent hypertension trial.[19] It is clear therefore by reference to Table 1.10 that the majority of non-smoking hypertensive

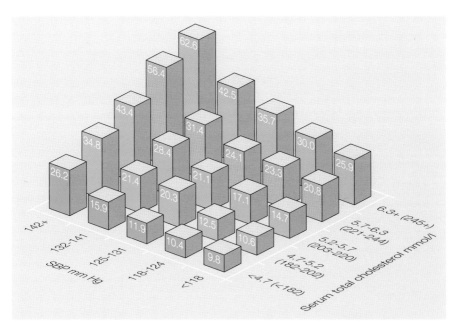

Fig. 1.14 Age-adjusted coronary heart disease death rates per 10,000 person-years by level of serum cholesterol and systolic BP for cigarette smokers screened in the Multiple Risk Factor Intervention Trial (rates per 10,000 person-years are noted on bars). (From Arch Intern Med 1992; 152: 56.)

patients (systolic BP $\geq$ 142 mmHg) are at an absolute risk of at least 2.3% in the next 10 years (22.69/10,000 person-years) of CHD death. The equivalent figure for smokers would be 5.6% in the next ten years. This puts the majority of non-smoking and smoking hypertensives at over 7-fold and 19-fold, respectively greater risk of CHD death compared with non-smokers with ideal systolic BP (< 118 mmHg) and 'ideal' cholesterol (< 182 mg %). This increased risk, along with that associated with low HDL cholesterol and raised triglycerides has implications for optimal intervention on lipid profiles in the hypertensive population (see Ch. 7, p. 96).

Summary

- Increasing levels of BP show a continuous graded relationship with cardiovascular risk.

- The pragmatic definition of hypertension is that level of BP above which investigation and treatment do more good than harm.

- Hypertension is one of the major contributors to the global burden of disease.

- The burden of disease due to raised BP is likely to worsen in the coming decades.

- In the western world the majority of adults over 50 years of age are considered hypertensive.

- The apparently inexorable rise in BP with age is actually largely preventable and hence so is hypertension.

References

1. Ezzati M, Lopez D, Rodgers A, Vander Hoom S, Murray CJ. Selected major risk factors and global and regional burden of disease. Lancet 2002; 360:1347–60.

2. Hypertension – a problem for the population. In: Bulpitt J (ed.) Epidemiology of Hypertension. Vol 20. Handbook of Hypertension. Elsevier Science BV, 2000.

3. Prospective Studies Collaboration. Age-specific relevance of usual blood pressure to vascular mortality: a meta-analysis of individual data for one million adults in 61 prospective studies. Lancet 2002; 350: 1903–13.

4. The JNC7 Report. The Seventh Report of the Joint National Committee on Prevention, Detection, Evaluation, and Treatment of High Blood Pressure. JAMA 2003; 289: 2560–72.

5. Guidelines Committee. 2003 European Society of Hypertension – European Society of Cardiology guidelines for the management of arterial hypertension. J Hypertens 2003; 21: 1011–53.

6. Primatesta P, Brookes M, Poulter NR. Improved hypertension management and control. Results from the Health Survey for England 1998. Hypertension 2001; 38: 827–832.

7. O'Rourke MF. From theory into practice. Arterial hemodynamics in clinical hypertension. J Hypertens 2002; 20: 1901–15.

8. Mancilha Carvalho JJ, Baruzzi RG, Howard PF et al. Blood pressure in four remote populations in the INTERSALT Study. Hypertension 1989; 14: 238–46.

9. Burt VL, Whelton P, Roccella EJ et al. Prevalence of hypertension in the US adult population. Results from the Third National Health and Nutrition Examination Survey, 1988–1991. Hypertension 1995; 25: 305–313.

10. Wolf-Maier K, Cooper RS, Banegas JR et al. Hypertension prevalence and blood pressure levels in 6 European countries, Canada, and the United States. JAMA 2003; 18: 2363–9.

11. Primatesta P, Bost L, Poulter NR. Blood pressure levels and hypertension status among ethnic groups in England. J Hum Hypertens 2000; 14: 143–8.

12. Hajjar I, Kotchen TA. Trends in prevalence, awareness, treatment, and control of hypertension in the United States, 1988–2000. JAMA 2003; 290: 199–206.

13. Amos et al. Diabetic Medicine 1997; 14: 57.

14. Reaven GM, Lithell H, Lansberg L. Hypertension and associated metablic abnormalities – the role of insulin resistance and the sympathoadrenal system. New Engl J Med 1996; 312: 406–10.

15. National Cholesterol Education Program. Third Report of the National Cholesterol Education Program (NCEP) Expert Panel on Detection, Evaluation, and Treatment of High Blood Cholesterol in Adults (Adult Treatment Panel III). Final report. Circulation 2002; 106: 3143–3421.

16. Poulter NR, Khaw KT, Hopwood BEC et al. The Kenyan Luo Migration Study: observations on the initiation of a rise in blood pressure. BMJ 1990; 300: 967–72.

17. Khaw KT, Barrett-Connor E. Dietary potassium and stroke-associated mortality. A 12 year prospective population study. N Engl J Med 1987; 316: 235–40.

18. Hanon O, Leys D. Cognitive decline and dementia in the elderly hypertensive. JRAAS 2002; 3: S32–38.

19. Sever PS, Dahlof B, Poulter NR et al. Rationale, design, methods and baseline demography of participants of the Anglo-Scandinavian Cardiac Outcomes Trial. J Hypertension 2001; 19: 1139–47.

Chapter 2

How should patients with hypertension be assessed?

The evaluation of a patient in relation to possible hypertension is initially aimed at establishing his or her real blood pressure (BP) levels. Thereafter the evaluation is aimed at identifying causes of raised BP and thereby possible targets for intervention and for estimating overall cardiovascular risk as a critical influence on intervention strategy.

Finally the identification of other coexisting conditions frequently influences management.

BP measurement

Accurate and reliable measurements of BP are critical to the diagnosis of hypertension – however defined – and to monitoring changes in BP levels in response to interventions and over time. BP varies dramatically within and between days and hence the diagnosis of hypertension is usually dependent on multiple BP recordings. Clearly the more marginal the BP evaluation, the more recordings are required over several months before therapy should be initiated, whereas more marked BP elevation with obvious target-organ damage requires fewer readings over a shorter timespan.

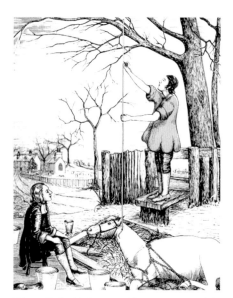

Fig. 2.1 Hales making manometric measurements from carotid artery of a horse in 1733.

BP measurements may be recorded in the clinic (or office) by the doctor or preferably the nurse, at home by the patient, or automatically over a 24-hour period (ambulatory blood pressure monitoring [ABPM]).

A working group of the European Society of Hypertension have recently published an extensive document outlining measurement procedures.[1] General guidelines for clinic or office readings are shown in Tables 2.1 and 2.2. Restriction of the use of mercury in Europe will increasingly impinge on the use of mercury sphygmomanometers. However replacement devices are limited in number and only those formally validated should be used.[2]

- Use device with validated accuracy, that is properly maintained and calibrated

- Measure sitting BP routinely: standing BP in elderly or diabetic patients

- Remove tight clothing, support arm at heart level, ensure hand relaxed, don't talk

- Use cuff of appropriate size (see Table 2.2)

- Lower mercury column slowly, by 2 mm per second

- Read BP to the nearest 2 mmHg

- Measure diastolic as disappearance of sounds (phase V)

- Take the mean of at least two readings; more recordings are needed if marked differences between initial measurements are found

- Use the average for several visits when estimating cardiovascular risk in mild hypertension

Table 2.1 BP measurement by standard mercury sphygmomanometer or semi-automated device

Indication	Bladder width × length (cm)	Arm circumference (cm)
Small adult/child	12 × 18	< 23
Standard adult	12 × 26	< 33
Large adult	12 ×40	< 50
Adult thigh cuff	20 × 42	< 53

Alternative adult cuffs (width × length, 12 × 35 cm) have been recommended for all adult patients but can result in problems with over- and undercuffing. The BHS recommends that cuff size be selected based on arm circumference.

Table 2.2 BP cuff sizes for mercury sphygmomanometer, semi-automatic and ambulatory monitors.

ABPM

Because of the natural variability of BP, ABPM recordings correlate better than clinic readings with target-organ damage and risk of cardiovascular events, and also tend to reduce the impact of white-coat hypertension.

Indications for ABPM are shown in Table 2.3 and some practical issues for the use of these devices are shown in Table 2.4.

Mean daytime and night-time ABPM values are usually used for assessment. Importantly these values are usually lower than clinic measurements and thresholds and targets should therefore be adjusted downwards (i.e. mean daytime levels using ABPM are roughly 10/5 mmHg lower than the equivalent clinic values).

- When BP shows unusual variability
- In excluding white-coat hypertension
- In helping with the assessment of patients with borderline hypertension
- In identifying nocturnal hypertension
- In assessing patients whose hypertension has been resistant to drug therapy (defined as BP > 150/90 mmHg on three or more anti-hypertensive drugs)
- As a guide to determining the efficacy of drug treatment over 24 hours
- In diagnosing and treating hypertension in pregnancy
- In diagnosing hypotension and postural hypotension
- To identify relation of BP levels to presumed side effects

Table 2.3 Potential indications for ABPM.

Home BP

Whilst repeat clinic BP measurement will, to an extent, offset the advantages of ABPM readings, those from home measurement are more likely to equate to those from ABPM. This method is relatively cheap and may improve adherence to therapy, but if used, readings should be taken over a period of a few days. This method should be discouraged among the proportion of patients who become anxious and obsessed with their BP readings. Some practical issues for the use of home monitoring include:[3]

- Only validated devices should be used. This currently excludes wrist devices.

- Semi-automatic devices are preferable as they are simpler to use than mercury sphygmomanometers.

- Seated measurements after several minutes of rest should be taken but warnings regarding spontaneous BP variability should be given.

- Limit the number of measurements taken, but if BP-lowering treatment is being taken, ensure a range of times are covered to evaluate peak and trough levels.

- As for ABPM, note that normal values are lower for home compared with office pressures. As a rough guide, take 130/85 mmHg at home as equivalent to 140/90 mmHg in the clinic.

- Clear instructions on how to document the measured values should be given, as should advice to avoid self-alteration of the treatment, unless pre-arranged.

- Use only validated devices

- Use appropriate cuff size (see Table 2.2)

- Advise patients to behave normally but avoid strenuous exercise

- Measure BP at 30-minute intervals during the day and hourly at night

- Keep arm extended and still during actual measurement

- Keep a diary of events during the day of measurement including duration and quality of sleep

- Repeat recording may be necessary if more than 30% of readings are artefactual

Table 2.4 Recommendations for device use.

Medical history

Most patients have no specific complaints regarding their raised BP. The critical questions that should be asked when taking a history are included in Table 2.5.

Examination

This should mainly be aimed at identifying signs of secondary causes of hypertension or more commonly signs of target-organ damage (Table 2.6). In addition other signs relating to cadiovascular risk (e.g. stigmata of unreported smoking or dyslipidaemia) should be picked up as should signs of potentially relevant coexisting conditions (e.g. asthma).

Investigations

These should be carried out with a view to evaluating possible causes of raised BP, the presence of target-organ damage and to allow an assessment of global cardiovascular risk. Recommendations regarding minimum tests required are relatively similar across three sets of recent guidelines[3-5] as shown in Table 2.7.

- Personal history
- Age
- Sex
- Smoking habits of patient
- Alcohol consumption
- Concomitant medication
- Physical activity
- Recreational drug usage
- Past and current history of coronary heart disease or cerebrovascular disease
- Diabetes
- Oral contraceptive use (and hormonal replacement therapy)
- Respiratory illness (especially asthma or chronic obstructive airways disease)
- Family history
- Past history of renal disease
- Past history of hypertension in pregnancy

Table 2.5 History taking.

Secondary hypertension		
	Enlarged kidneys (polycystic kidneys)	
	Delayed radio-femoral pulsation (coarctation)	
	Neurofibromatosis (phaeochromocytoma)	
	Cushing's syndrome	
	Alcohol excess (e.g. liver palms, tremor, etc.)	
	Abdominal bruits (renal artery stenosis)	
Target-organ damage		
	Displaced apex (LVH)	
	Arterial bruits (carotid, femoral)	
	Absent peripheral pulses (PAD)	
	Heart failure (third heart sound, raised JVP etc.)	
	Hypertensive retinopathy	
	Arrhythmia	

Table 2.6 Signs of secondary causes of hypertension and target-organ damage.

Global risk assessment

Rationale

The aetiology of coronary heart disease (CHD) and stroke have been known for decades to be multifactorial.[6] Increasing risk of both CHD and stroke has been shown to have a graded continuous relationship with increasing BP across the whole BP range.[7] Furthermore among the hypertensive population, however defined, the coexistence of other risk factors such as age, smoking, and cholesterol have been shown to result in a dramatic increase in risk associated with any BP stratum. Consequently the absolute risk of a cardiovascular event occurring in hypertensive patients varies dramatically, perhaps more than 20-fold, depending on age, sex, level of BP, and on the coexistence of other risk factors.[8]

The JNC 6 guidelines from the USA introduced a crude risk classification method to guide treatment thresholds.[9] Patients are classified into one

BHS
- Urine test strip (protein and blood)
- Se. creatinine and electrolytes
- Fasting glucose
- Fasting lipid profile (total, HDL and TGs)
- ECG
- Uric acid

ESH-ESC
Routine tests:
- Plasma glucose (preferably fasting)
- Serum total cholesterol
- Serum HDL cholesterol
- Fasting serum triglycerides
- Serum uric acid
- Serum creatinine
- Serum potassium
- Haemoglobin and haematocrit
- Urinalysis (dipstick test complemented by urinary sediment examination)
- Electrocardiogram

Recommended tests:
- ECG
- Carotid (and femoral) ultrasound
- C-reactive protein
- Microalbuminuria (essential test in diabetics)
- Quantitative proteinuria (if dipstick test positive)
- Fundoscopy (in severe hypertension)

JNC 7
Routine laboratory tests recommended before initiating therapy:
- ECG
- Urinalysis
- Blood glucose and hematocrit
- Serum potassium, creatinine (or the corresponding estimated glomerular filtration rate), and calcium and a lipid profile (after a 9–12-hour fast that includes HDL cholesterol, low-density lipoprotein (LDL) cholesterol, and triglycerides

Optional tests:
- Measurement of urinary albumin excretion or albumin/creatinine ratio

*More extensive testing for identifiable causes is not indicated generally unless BP control is not achieved.

Table 2.7 Recent guidelines for recommended minimum tests required*.

of three categories of coexistent risk factors (from nil to established disease or target-organ damage) for each of three or four grades of BP. One study did confirm that, despite its crude nature, this approach did differentiate those at highest risk from those at less risk.[10] This type of risk stratification was subsequently adopted by the World Health Organisation/International Society of Hypertension (WHO–ISH) guidelines produced in 1999[11] and in their follow-up statement in 2003.[12] Interestingly however in an apparently retrogressive move, in the most recent JNC 7 guidelines no mention of risk stratification is made.[5]

Several other more complex and accurate methods of predicting relatively short-term risk of either a CHD event or a cardiovascular event (stroke or CHD) have been developed.[13–15] The most commonly used risk scores have arisen from the algorithm derived from the Framingham cohort,[15] and in relation to coronary rather than cardiovascular risk. Several established risk factors are not included in the risk scores, in part for logistical reasons (risk charts cannot include more than a few variables) and also because the original cohort studies which provided the risk assessment databases did not measure some of the factors which clearly do impact independently on risk.

The exclusion of risk factors such as pulse rate,[16] microalbuminuria,[17] exercise,[18] high sensitivity crp,[19] and migraine,[20] inevitably means that at the individual level, risk scores may be significantly inaccurate. Furthermore the risk associated with some of the risk factors, such as smoking or diabetes, may be miscalculated because they are treated dichotomously – present or absent. This results in inaccuracy and misclassification because it is clear that, in the case of diabetes, the risk associated with glycaemia, as assessed by HbA1C level, is graded and continuous[21] and the level of risk is further affected by duration of the diagnosis. Similarly, regarding smoking-related risk, a person who has smoked one cigarette per day for the last 2 years may be classified as a smoker, whereas someone who stopped smoking 5 years ago, having smoked 60 cigarettes per day for 30 years, may be considered a non-smoker. Such classification will inevitably produce inaccurate results.

In summary, all risk assessment tools, by virtue of limited and misclassified variables, are inevitably inaccurate and should only provide guidance in the context of all the available information gleaned from a thorough medical investigation.

Despite the shortcomings of the Framingham database – a relatively small, mainly white, middle class cohort from Massachusetts, USA – the score it produces has been shown to be reasonably accurate when applied to the northern European setting.[22] Its generalisibility to southern Europe and other ethnic subgroups however is less clear.

Nevertheless early European guidelines produced a chart to help evaluate risk of developing CHD based on Framingham.[23] By including high-density lipoprotein (HDL) cholesterol these charts were improved upon in New Zealand guidelines whose charts could be used to estimate the 5-year risk of a cardiovascular rather than a CHD event.[24]

These charts were refined and simplified, and incorporated into the Joint British Recommendations, although this group, for reasons of consistency with European and Scottish guidelines, reverted to evaluating coronary risk.[25] This chart, like all of the others of its kind, has one consistent and important inherent problem: that is that they predict short-term (usually 5- or 10-year) absolute risk, which is used as a key determinant of intervention (or not). This causes undertreatment of young people at high relative risk and overtreatment of older people at lower relative risk. For example, a 32-year-old woman, even if she is diabetic, a smoker, has a total cholesterol:HDL ratio of 8, and a systolic BP of 170 mmHg, does not reach a 10-year risk of CHD of 30% – the threshold at which intervention has been recommended for some therapies. In contrast, most elderly men (e.g. those aged 70) would reach this risk level and hence qualify for intervention simply on account of their age and sex. The European approach to offset this problem was to 'project' young people with high levels of risk factors to age 60 and to base treatment decisions on the resulting estimated level of risk. This is one way of reducing the ageism and sexism inherent in current risk assessment charts.

The Joint British Recommendations in 1998 produced a user-friendly computerised risk assessor that included a larger number of variables than in their chart and hence provided a more accurate risk calculation for both CHD and stroke.[25] However of the nine variables included in the risk assessor, three of them – smoking, diabetes, and left ventricular hypertrophy (LVH) on electrocardiogram (ECG) are dealt with dichotomously with all the shortcomings of such an approach described earlier.

It should be noted that the Framingham risk equation which underpins all of these charts related not only to fatal CHD and non-fatal myocardial infarction (AMI), but also silent myocardial infarction (MI) and 'coronary insufficiency' – presumably equivalent to unstable angina. Conscious of criticism that this score overpredicted risk in certain situations, a new score was produced in the National Cholesterol Education Program, ATP III report, based on 'harder' end-points - fatal CHD and stroke, and non-fatal MI and stroke.[26]

In clinical practice however both the prescribing doctor and patient are likely to be interested in all major cardiovascular events including stroke and heart failure, and procedures such as angioplasty and bypass grafting, rather than just fatal and non-fatal CHD, and certainly not just fatal events.

The most recent risk score produced in Europe is that which has emerged from the SCORE project.[27] Based on 12 European cohort studies—most but not all of which are population based—including about 2.7 million years of follow up, a chart or computer-based system of predicting stroke or CHD death ('cardiovascular death') has been developed. Acknowledging the important impact of differences in background rates of cardiovascular death, risk estimation charts have been produced for high and low cardiovascular event populations, with or without the inclusion of HDL cholesterol. The latter modification reflects major differences of opinion within Europe regarding the importance of HDL cholesterol in risk calculation, not to mention its availability as a routine measure. The authors of the SCORE project report no effect of the inclusion or exclusion of HDL in their risk prediction model, whilst counter-arguments propose that this reflects different and inadequate measurements of HDL in the various studies that generated the database.

One clear advantage of the computerised version of the SCORE system is the ability to incorporate whatever additional 'favourite' risk factor the user may wish as an extra dimension.

The major downside to this system is that the outcome measure – cardiovascular death – is not the one which patients and doctors are most concerned about. Furthermore the charts are complicated (Fig. 2.2) and incorporate a new range of numbers that physicians (who are only just getting to grips with 10-year CHD risk thresholds of 15%, 20% or 30%) are likely to find confusing.

A further problem with the SCORE system is that diabetic subjects were included at baseline in the databases of the cohorts used, and results cannot be differentiated for diabetic and non-diabetic subjects. The recommendation for calculating risk in diabetic subjects using this method therefore is to double the estimate calculated for males and quadruple that estimated for females. This seems very crude and probably provides little, if anything, over Framingham-based calculations with the associated well-established limitations of this algorithm due to small numbers of diabetic subjects.

The need for risk estimation among diabetic subjects is, in itself, controversial. In the most recent Adult Treatment Panel III (ATPIII) report[28] the recommendation is to consider those with type 2 diabetes as 'coronary equivalents', thereby obviating the need for risk assessment. This is based on one Finnish study[29] that conflicts with other epidemiological data.[30] However, the evidence strongly suggests that the CHD risk among diabetic subjects aged older than 50, or those who have been diagnosed for at least 10 years, is equivalent to that which post-MI patients are exposed. Furthermore the short (1 month) and long (1 year) term case–fatality rates for patients with diabetes is much higher than for those without. Hence for simplicity, given that most patients with type 2 diabetes are aged over 50, it seems reasonable to treat this group as coronary equivalents, which in turn pre-empts the need for global risk estimation. However a risk scoring system ('engine') has been developed, based on the UK Prospective Diabetes Study Group (UKPDS) trial, for patients with diabetes.[31] Whilst this is undoubtedly a more accurate tool for assessing diabetic risk than any other method available, its value may be restricted to the small number of patients aged younger than 50 years who have not been diabetic for 10 years or more.

The ideal requirements of a risk factor scoring system tend to contradict each other. For example, to be valid, a score needs to be comprehensive, which pre-empts the requirements of simplicity, inexpensiveness and user-friendliness.

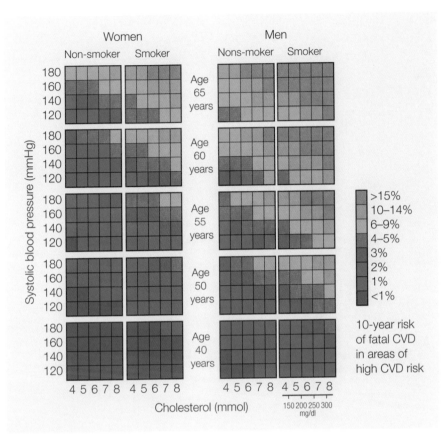

Fig. 2.2 SCORE project.

Nevertheless, the JNC 7 recommendations notwithstanding, assessment of global risk is increasingly endorsed and encouraged as a guide to clinical practice, and strategies that do not incorporate such an approach are likely to be less cost-effective and/or affordable overall.

The trade-off between accuracy and simplicity can only be ultimately overcome by computerised systems, which incorporate many more variables. This assumes that data on all these variables are likely to become routinely collected. Meanwhile the ideal system should predict all major cardiovascular (rather than coronary) events (not just fatal ones) and incorporate some method of avoiding the shortcomings of predicting only short-term absolute risk. To date, admittedly with more emphasis on simplicity than accuracy, the charts due to be produced in the next iteration of the British Hypertension Society Guidelines[4] and the Joint British Recommendations[32] will be the best available option. This tool, like all of the others available, should be used to guide rather than rule practice by clinicians, who should be fully aware of the shortcomings of the system in use.

Summary

Optimal assessment of raised BP involves:

- Careful and acurate BP measurement using standardise procedures.

- Evaluation of causes of raised BP and hence targets for intervention.

- Assessment of overall cardiovascular risk.

- Identification of other coexisting conditions.

References

1. O'Brien E, Asmar R, Beilin L et al on behalf of the European Society of Hypertension Working Group on Blood Pressure Monitoring. European Society of Hypertension recommendations for conventional, ambulatory and home blood pressure measurement. J Hyertens 2003; 21: 821–48.

2. British Hypertension Society. Validated blood pressure monitors. http://www.bhsoc.org/

3. Guidelines Committee. 2003 European Society of Hypertension – European Society of Cardiology guidelines for the management of arterial hypertension. J Hypertens 2003; 21: 1011–53.

4. Bryan Williams, Neil R Poulter, Morris J Brown, Mark Davis, Gordon T McInnes, John F Potter, Peter S Sever, and Simon McG Thom. British Hypertension Society guidelines for hypertension management 2004 (BHS-IV): summary. BMJ 2004;328:634-640.

5. The JNC7 Report. The Seventh Report of the Joint National Committee on Prevention, Detection, Evaluation, and Treatment of High Blood Pressure. JAMA 2003; 289: 2560–72.

6. Labarthe DR. Atherosclerosis. In: Labarthe DR (ed.) Epidemiology and Prevention of Cardiovascular Diseases: A Global Challenge. Aspen Publishers Inc., 1998

7. Prospective Studies Collaboration. Age-specific relevance of usual blood pressure to vascular mortality: a meta-analysis of individual data for one million adults in 61 prospective studies. Lancet 2002; 360: 1903–13.

8. Stamler J. Established major coronary risk factors. In: Marmot M, Elliott P (eds) Coronary Heart Disease Epidemiology: from Aetiology to Public Health. Oxford: Oxford Medical Publications, 1992:

9. Joint National Committee on Prevention, Detection, Evaluation, and Treatment of High Blood Pressure. The sixth report of the Joint National Committee on Prevention, Detection, Evaluation and Treatment of High Blood Pressure. Arch Intern Med 1997; 157: 2413–46.

10. Ogden LG, He J, Lydick E, Whelton, PK. Long-term absolute benefit of lowering blood pressure in hypertensive patients according to the JNC VI Risk Stratification. Hypertension 2000; 34: 539–43.

11. Guidelines Subcommittee. 1999 World Health Organization-International Society of Hypertension Guidelines for the Management of Hypertension. J Hypertens 1999; 17: 151–83.

12. World Health Organization-International Society of Hypertension Writing Group 2003. World Health Organization (WHO)–International Society of Hypertension (ISH) Statement on management of hypertension. J Hypertens 2003; 21: 1983–92.

13. Shaper AG, Pocock SJ, Philips AN, Walker M. Identifying men at high risk of heart attacks: strategy for use in general practice. Br Med J 1986: 293; 474–9.

14. Assman G, Cullen P, Schulte H. Simple scoring scheme for calculating the risk of acute coronary events based on the 1-year follow-up of the prospective cardiovascular Munster (PROCAM) study. Circulation 2002; 105: 310–15.

15. Anderson KM, Wilson PW, Odell PM, Kannel WB. An updated coronary risk profile: a statement for health professionals. Circulation 1991; 83: 356–62.

16. Shaper AG, Wannamethee G, Macfarlane PW, Walker M. Heart rate, ischaemic heart disease, and sudden cardiac death in middle-aged British men. Br Heart J 1993; 70: 49–55.

17. Miettinen H, Haffner SM, Lehto S, Ronnemaa , Pyorala K, Laakso M. Proteinuria predicts stroke and other atherosclerotic vascular disease events in nondiabetic and non-insulin-dependent diabetic subjects. Stroke 1996; 27: 2033–39.

18. National Institutes of Health Consensus Development Program. Physical activity and cardiovascular health. NIH Consensus Statement 1995 December 18–20; 13(3): 1–33.

19. Ridker PM. High-sensitivity C-reactive protein: Potential adjunct for global risk assessment in the primary prevention of cardiovascular disease. Circulation 2001; 103: 1813–18.

20. Chang CL, Donaghy M, Poulter NR. Migraine and stroke in young women: a case–control study. Br Med J 1999; 318: 13–18.

21. Khaw KT, Wareham N, Luben R, Bingham S, Oakes S, Welch A. Glycated haemoglobin, diabetes, and mortality in men in Norfolk cohort of European Prospective Investigation of Cancer and Nutrition (EPIC-NORFOLK). Br Med J 2001; 322: 15–18.

22. Haq IU, Ramsay LE, Yeo WW, Jackson PR, Wallis EJ. Is the Framingham risk function valid for northern European populations? A comparison of methods for estimating absolute coronary risk in high risk men. Heart 1999; 81: 40–46.

23. Pyorala K, De Backer G, Graham I, Poole-Wilson P, Wood D on behalf of the Task Force. Prevention of coronary heart disease in clinical practice. Recommendations of the Task Force of the European Society of Cardiology, European Atherosclerosis Society and European Society of Hypertension. Eur Heart J 1994; 110: 121–61; International Society of Hypertension News 1995; 1: 6–12.

24. Jackson R. Updated New Zealand cardiovascular disease risk–benefit prediction guide. Br Med J 2000; 320: 709–10.

25. Wood D, Durrington P, Poulter N, McInnes G, Rees A, Wray R for the British Cardiac Society, British Hyperlipidaemia Association, British Hypertension Society, and British Diabetic Association. Joint British recommendations on prevention of coronary heart disease in clinical practice. Heart 1998; 80: S1–29.

26. Anonymous. Third Report of the National Cholesterol Education Program (NCEP) Expert Panel on Detection, Evaluation, and Treatment of High Blood Cholesterol in Adults (Adult Treatment Panel III) final report. Circulation 2002; 106: 3143–3421.

27. Conroy RM, Pyorala K, Fitzgerald AP et al on behalf of the SCORE project group. Estimation of ten-year risk of fatal cardiovascular disease in Europe: the SCORE project. Eur Heart J 2003; 24: 987–1003.

28. Executive Summary of the Third report of the National Cholesterol Education Program (NCEP) Expert Panel on detection, evaluation,

and treatment of high blood cholesterol in adults (Adult Treatment Panel III). JAMA 2001; 285: 2486–97.

29. Haffner SM, Lehto S, Ronnemaa T, Pyorala K, Laakso M. Mortality from coronary heart disease in subjects with type 2 diabetes and in nondiabetic subjects with and without prior myocardial infarction. New Engl J Med 1998; 339: 229–34.

30. Evans JMM, Wang J, Morris AD. Comparison of cardiovascular risk between patients with type 2 diabetes and those who had a myocardial infarction: cross sectional and cohort studies. Br Med J 2002; 324: 939–43.

31. UKPDS Group. The UKPDS Risk Engine: a model for the risk of coronary heart disease in type 2 diabetes (UKPDS 56). Clin Sci 2001; 101: 671–9.

32. Wood D, Durrington P, Poulter N et al. Joint British Societies Guidelines for CVD Prevention (in press).

Chapter 3

At what level should drug treatment be initiated?

The response to this question is best dealt with by considering patients on the basis of their cardiovascular risk status.

Patients at < 20% risk of a major cardiovascular event in the next 10 years

In this type of patient, evidence of the benefits of initiating drug therapy to lower blood pressure (BP) at thresholds less than 160 mmHg systolic are limited to observational data. Some evidence from early randomised, placebo-controlled trials did support an intervention threshold of 90 mmHg diastolic BP, but the most robust data from trials overall confirmed the benefits of treatment at levels of 160 mmHg systolic and above or 100 mmHg diastolic and above.[1] While there has been no new clinical trial evidence to support lowering thresholds to below 160 mmHg systolic and 90 mmHg diastolic in hypertensive patients at low risk, recent observational data[2,3] do support earlier data[4] that suggest that systolic thresholds below 160 mmHg may be appropriate. These observational data suggest that even low-risk patients (< 15% 10-year cardiovascular risk) with BP $\geq$ 140 mmHg systolic and/or $\geq$ 90 mmHg diastolic are likely to benefit from lower pressures. Guidelines do not differentiate between men and women regarding optimal thresholds, although women are at lower absolute risk of cardiovascular disease for a given level of BP than men, and randomised, controlled trial (RCT) evidence includes a greater proportion of men than women.

Although the absolute risk of cardiovascular diseases for any given level of BP rises with age, only limited RCT evidence is currently available about the benefits of treating those over 80 years of age. Hence, pending further data, the treatment threshold should be unaffected by age at least up to the age of 80 years. Thereafter, decisions should be made ad personem but therapy should not be withdrawn from patients over 80 years of age purely on the basis of age.

Patients with established vascular disease or at high risk of developing it (> 20% 10-year cardiovascular risk)

Several recently published trials in high-risk patients[5-8] have shown morbidity and mortality benefits associated with lowering BPs from thresholds significantly below 160 mmHg systolic and/or 90 mmHg diastolic. These trials, details of which are discussed in Chapter 6, p. 87, show that irrespective of initial BP, additional BP lowering in high-risk patients results in a significant reduction in cardiovascular event rates. Similarly other smaller trials evaluating the effect of angiotensin II receptor blockers (ARBs) on the progression of diabetic nephropathy also suggest that treatment for such patients should begin at lower thresholds.[9–11]

Figures 3.1–3.3 show the algorithms provided in three sets of recent guidelines from the UK,[12] USA,[13] and Europe[14] regarding when to initiate non-pharmcological and drug treatment to lower BP.

In the UK and European sets of guidelines, but not JNC 7, the initiation of an intervention is dependent not only on the level of systolic and/ or diastolic pressure, but to one extent or another also involves some

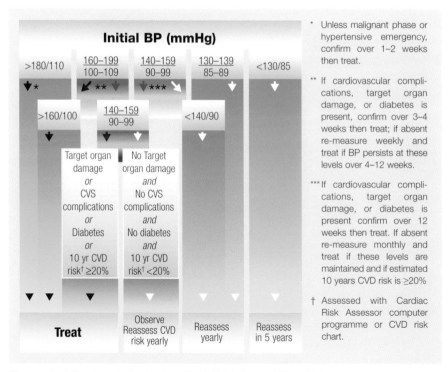

Figure 3.1 Treatment thresholds: BHS Guidelines 1999/2004.

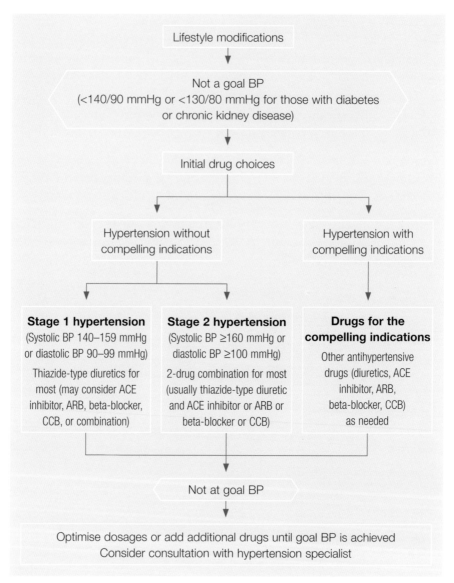

Figure 3.2 Algorithm for treatment of hypertension: JNC 7.[13]

estimation of total (global) cardiovascular risk. One apparent anomaly incorporated into all three sets of guidelines (and most previous similar documents) is the allegiance of a systolic BP of 140 mmHg with a diastolic BP of 90 mmHg. In reality, whether in the general population or among

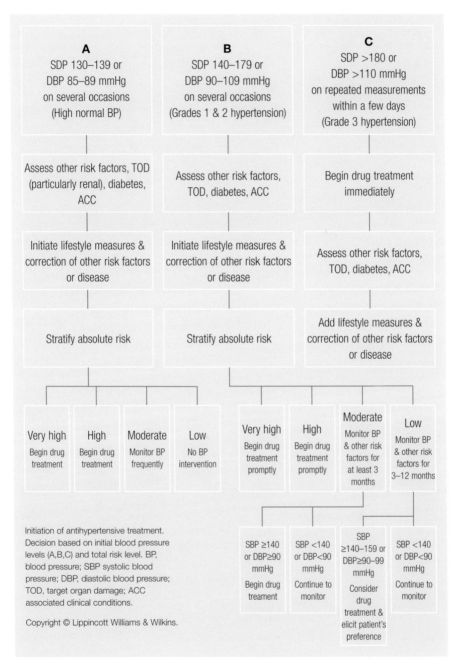

A
SDP 130–139 or
DBP 85–89 mmHg
on several occasions
(High normal BP)

B
SDP 140–179 or
DBP 90–109 mmHg
on several occasions
(Grades 1 & 2 hypertension)

C
SDP >180 or
DBP >110 mmHg
on repeated measurements
within a few days
(Grade 3 hypertension)

Assess other risk factors, TOD
(particularly renal), diabetes,
ACC

Assess other risk factors,
TOD, diabetes, ACC

Begin drug treatment
immediately

Initiate lifestyle measures &
correction of other risk factors
or disease

Initiate lifestyle measures &
correction of other risk factors
or disease

Assess other risk factors,
TOD, diabetes, ACC

Stratify absolute risk

Stratify absolute risk

Add lifestyle measures &
correction of other risk factors
or disease

Very high
Begin drug
treatment

High
Begin drug
treatment

Moderate
Monitor BP
frequently

Low
No BP
intervention

Very high
Begin drug
treatment
promptly

High
Begin drug
treatment
promptly

Moderate
Monitor BP
& other risk
factors for
at least 3
months

Low
Monitor BP
& other risk
factors for
3–12 months

SBP ≥140
or DBP≥90
mmHg

Begin drug
treament

SBP <140
or DBP<90
mmHg

Continue to
monitor

SBP
≥140–159 or
DBP≥90–99
mmHg

Consider
drug
treatment &
elicit patient's
preference

SBP <140
or DBP<90
mmHg

Continue to
monitor

Initiation of antihypertensive treatment.
Decision based on initial blood pressure
levels (A,B,C) and total risk level. BP,
blood pressure; SBP systolic blood
pressure; DBP, diastolic blood pressure;
TOD, target organ damage; ACC
associated clinical conditions.

Copyright © Lippincott Williams & Wilkins.

Figure 3.3 Treatment threshold algorithm: ESH-ESC guidelines.[14]

Months	SBP (mmHg)	DBP (mmHg)
0	162.3	92.4
1.5	151.5	85.6
3	146.7	83.5
6	144.4	83.4
12	141.6	82.0
18	138.7	79.8
24	137.8	80.1
30	136.0	78.7

Table 3.1 Mean BP's of over 9000 patients recruited and followed up in a hypertension trial.

treated hypertensive patients (except possibly in young adults), these two levels are not compatible in the vast majority of people (see Tables 1.2 and 3.1). In short, as seen in these two datasets, if the systolic BP is less than 140 mmHg, the diastolic BP will almost invariably be much less than 90 mmHg.

A further consistent shortcoming in all these guidelines is their complexity. In an era of ever-increasing guideline production in scores of different areas of medicine, the lack of simplicity for the practising physician may be a genuine and important barrier to implementation of the recommendations included (see Ch. 9, p. 111).

Variations in guidance

The major difference between these sets of guidance is that the BHS recommendations are more conservative. The European and US recommendations effectively suggest that all adults with a systolic BP of ≥ 140 mmHg after some attempt at non-pharmacological intervention will merit drug treatment for raised BP, whereas the BHS guidelines restrict drug use to those above a specified level of risk. Whilst by European recommendations, such a person needs one other risk factor to merit drug treatment, it is clear from the wide range of qualifying variables that the vast majority of subjects do have at least one of the qualifying risk factors.[14] The American approach is even more aggressive in that no such additional risk factor is required to merit drug intervention.

The impact of these recommendations, if implicated, on the use of antihypertensive medication and the associated workload is likely to be huge since, in England for example, about three-quarters of all adults aged 65 or older have a systolic BP of at least 140 mmHg.[15] Whilst it is most likely that mass treatment with antihypertensive medication of almost all those in this age group (by virtue of 140/90 criteria) will produce benefit in terms of reducing cardiovascular events, no trial evidence is available to confirm the likelihood of such benefits except for those at high risk.[5-8] Furthermore it is conceptually wrong that we accept such a fate as normal for almost all those aged 65 years and older. This situation can only be avoided by a population-based preventive strategy to stop or attenuate the rise of BP throughout adult life, hitherto considered inevitable in westernised society (see Ch. 1, p. 5).

Summary

- Guidence re. thresholds for intervention is frequently beyond supportive trial evidence.

- For many patients evaluation of total CV risk is required to determine whether to treat with drugs or not.

- The British Hypertension Society thresholds are recommended (see Fig 3.1).

References

1. Collins R, Peto R, MacMahon S et al. Blood pressure, stroke, and coronary heart disease. Part 2, Short-term reductions in blood pressure: overview of randomised drug trials in their epidemiological context. Lancet 1990; 335: 827–29.

2. Van den Hoogen PCW, Feskens EJM, Nagelkerke NJD, Menotti A, Nissinen A, Kromhout D for the Seven Countries Study Research Group. The relation between blood pressure and mortality due to coronary heart disease among men in different parts of the world. N Engl J Med 2000; 342: 1–8.

3. Vasan RS, Larson MG, Leip EP et al. Impact of high-normal pressure on the risk of cardiovascular disease. N Engl J Med 2001; 345: 1291–7.

4. MacMahon S, Peto R, Cutler J et al. Blood pressure, stroke, and coronary heart disease. Part 1, Prolonged differences in blood pressure: prospective observational studies corrected for the regression dilution bias. Lancet 1990; 335: 765–74.

5. The Heart Outcomes Prevention Evaluation Study Investigators. Effects of an angiotensin-converting-enzyme inhibitor, ramipril, on cardiovascular events in high-risk patients. N Engl J Med 2000; 342: 145–53.

6. PROGRESS Collaborative Study Group. Randomised trial of perindopril based blood pressure-lowering regimen among 6108 individuals with previous stroke or transient ischaemic attack. Lancet 2001; 358: 1033–41.

7. The EURopean trial On reduction of cardiac events with Perindopril in stable coronary Artery disease investigators. Efficacy of perindopril in reduction of cardiovascular events among patients with stable coronary artery disease: randomised, double-blind, placebo-controlled, multicentre trial (the EUROPA study). Lancet 2003; 362: 782–8.

8. Lithell H, Hansson L, Skoog I, Elmfeldt D, Hofman A, Olofsson B, Trenkwalder P, Zanchetti A for the SCOPE Study Group. The Study

on Cognition and Prognosis in the Elderly (SCOPE): principal results of a randomized double-blind intervention trial. J Hypertens 2003; 21: 875–86.

9. Lewis EJ, Hunsicker LG, Clarke WR et al. Renoprotective effect of the angiotensin-receptor antagonist irbesartan in patients with nephropathy due to type 2 diabetes. N Engl J Med 2001; 345: 851–60.

10. Parving HH, Lehnert H, Brochner-Mortensen J, Gomis R, Andersen S, Arner P. The effect of irbesartan on the development of diabetic nephropathy in patients with type 2 diabetes. N Engl J Med 2001; 345: 870–8.

11. Brenner BM, Cooper ME, De Zeeuw D et al. Effects of losartan on renal and cardiovascular outcomes in patients with type 2 diabetes and nephropathy. N Engl J Med 2001; 345: 861–9.

12. Ramsay LE, Williams B, Johnston GD et al. Guidelines for Management of Hypertension: Report of the third working party of the British Hypertension Society, 1999. J Human Hypertens 1999; 13: 569–92.

13. The JNC7 Report. The Seventh Report of the Joint National Committee on Prevention, Detection, Evaluation, and Treatment of High Blood Pressure. JAMA 2003; 289: 2560–72.

14. Guidelines Committee. 2003 European Society of Hypertension-European Soceity of Cardiology guidelines for the management of arterial hypertension. J Hypertens 2003; 21: 1011–53.

15. Primatesta P, Poulter NR. Hypertension management and control among English adults aged 65 years and older in 2000 and 2001. J Hypertens 2004;22:1093-1098.

Chapter 4

Is non-drug treatment worthwhile?

Although the benefits of non-phamacological manoeuvres are by no means established across the whole blood pressure (BP) range above 'normal' or optimal (i.e. > 120 mmHg systolic or > 80 mmHg diastolic BP) the lifestyle changes recommended in all recent sets of guidelines for hypertension management are likely to benefit the whole of society, irrespective of BP level. At the very worst these changes are deemed harmless. Nevertheless it must be admitted that the extensive trial evidence relating to non-drug measures, which does exist, is almost exclusively in relation to benefits in terms of BP lowering or deferring the development of hypertension rather than on the prevention of major cardiovascular events.

One area of confusion that appears to pervade the area of lifestyle interventions is that relating to the interpretation of the efficacy of such manoeuvres. In studies, admittedly of short duration in most cases, in which compliance with dietary interventions is achieved (e.g. reduction of fat intake to lower cholesterol), benefits on risk factors (e.g. blood lipid levels) have clearly been shown. However when compliance with dietary manoeuvres has not been achieved, no benefits have accrued. Based on the intention-to-treat principle this has been misinterpreted to mean that diets 'don't work'. A more realistic summary of the situation is that the ability of health professionals to persuade patients to change their diets and lifestyles is limited. However if and when healthy lifestyle manoeuvres are taken up, benefits, albeit on surrogate end-points, do seem to accrue.

Evidence

The lifestyle modifications and supportive references that have been shown in clinical trials to lower BP or reduce the incidence of hypertension are shown in Table 4.1.

Extensive investigation and controversy surrounds other lifestyle measures not included in Table 4.1, but overall it appears that calcium[9] and magnesium supplements,[10] reduction in caffeine intake[11] and various stress-reducing techniques[12] do not produce significant or lasting beneficial effects on BP levels.

To reduce BP:

- Weight reduction[1,2]

- Dietary sodium reduction[3-5]

- Moderation of alcohol intake[6]

- Increase fresh fruit and vegetable intake[3]

- Reduce saturated fat intake[3]

- Increase physical activity[7]

To reduce cardiovascular risk:

- Stop smoking

- Reduce total and saturated fat intake

- Increase fish consumption

Table 4.1 Recommended lifestyle interventions

Whilst smoking causes acute rises in BP and pulse rate, the effect of smoking (except possibly chronic heavy smoking) on BP is probably insignificant.[8]

Nevertheless, because of the acute effects of smoking on BP, the practical implication of BP measures taken whilst not smoking is to systematically underestimate the systolic BP of a smoker by about 10 mmHg compared with when he or she is actually smoking. For a smoker of 15 cigarettes per day, for example, this understated adverse effect on BP will last for about 7.5 hours per day!

Finally, given the frequent coexistence of hypertension in patients with type II diabetes, it is important to note the findings of two major trials[13,14] that have shown the benefits of diet and lifestyle interventions (including weight control) with a low-fat, low-calorie diet, and increase in exercise output and dietary fibre intake on the incidence of the development of type 2 diabetes among those with impaired glucose tolerance. In addition several dietary studies have shown the beneficial effects of fat restriction and exercise output on lipid levels.[15] Given the frequent coexistence of dyslipidaemia in hypertension (see Ch. 1, p. 21) the value of these manoeuvres for the overall benefit of patients with hypertension seem clear.

Non-drug measures and antihypertensive medication

Overall best evidence suggests that most non-drug measures are at least additive, in terms of BP lowering, to the effects of antihypertensive medication. However weight loss is made more difficult in the face of beta-blockers[16] and salt restriction may be marginally less effective when used in combination with a diuretic. On the other hand the effect of salt restriction, by priming the renin–angiotensin system, would be predicted to have a more than additive BP-lowering effect when used in combination with ACE inhibitors and angiotensin II receptor blockers (ARBs).

Summary

- Lifestyle modifications recommended in all recent guidelines for patients with hypertension should probably be adopted at a population level by all individuals, irrespective of BP level.

- If implicated, this would be expected to have a massive beneficial impact on cardiovascular outcomes[17] and would, over two generations, be likely to reduce if not greatly attenuate the usual rise of BP with age experienced in westernised populations.

- Lifestyle modifications would have a dramatic impact on the high prevalence of hypertension which is accepted as 'the norm' in industrialised populations.

- The uptake of these manoeuvres by the population with less than ideal BPs would reduce the number of people progressing to need antihypertensive medication, and among those who still need antihypertensive drugs, the average dosage and/or number of drugs used would be reduced.

References

1. Stevens VJ, Obarzanek E, Cook NR et al. Long-term weight loss and changes in results of the Trials of Hypertension Prevention, Phase II. Ann Intern Med 2001; 134: 1–11.

2. Leiter LA, Abbott D, Campbell NRC, Mendelson R, Ogilvie RI, Chockalingam. A recommendation on obesity and weight loss. CMAJ 1999; 160(Suppl 9): S7–11.

3. Sacks FM, Svetkey LP, Vollmer WM et al. Third Effects on blood pressure of reduced dietary sodium and the Dietary Approaches to Stop Hypertension (DASH) diet. DASH Sodium Collaborative Research Group. N Engl J Med 2001; 344: 3–10.

4. Cutler JA, Follmann D, Allender PS. Randomized trials of sodium reduction: An overview. Am J Clin Nutr 1997; 65(Suppl): 643S–51S.

5. Whelton PK, Appel LJ, Espeland MA et al. Sodium reduction and weight loss in the treatment of hypertension in older persons: A randomized controlled trial of non-pharmacological interventions in the elderly (TONE). JAMA 1998; 279: 839–46.

6. Xin X, He J, Frontini MG, Ogden LG, Motsamai OI, Whelton PK. Effects of alcohol reduction on blood pressure: A meta-analysis of randomized controlled trials. Hypertension 2001; 38: 1112–7.

7. Hagberg JM, Park JJ, Brown MD. The role of exercise training in the treatment of hypertension: An update. Sports Med 2000; 30: 193–206.

8. Primatesta P, Falaschetti E, Gupta S, Marmot MG, Poulter NR. Association between smoking and blood pressure. Evidence from the Health Survey for England. Hypertension 2001; 37: 187–93.

9. Griffith LE, Guyatt GH, Cook RJ, Bucher HC, Cook DJ. The influence of dietary and non-dietary calcium supplementation on blood pressure. An updated meta-analysis of randomized controlled trials. Am J Hypertens 1999; 12: 84–92.

10. Kawano Y, Matsuoka H, Takishita S, Omae T. Effects of magnesium supplementation in hypertensive patients. Assessment by office, home, and ambulatory blood pressures. Hypertension 1998; 32: 260–265

11. Jee SH, He J, Whelton PK, Suh I, Klag MJ. The effect of chronic coffee drinking on blood pressure. A meta-analysis of controlled clinical trials. Hypertension 1999; 33: 647–652.

12. Spence JD, Barnett PA, Linden W, Ramsden V, Taenzer P. Lifestyle modifications to prevent and control hypertension. Recommendations on stress management. CMAJ 1999; 160(Suppl 9): S46–50.

13. Tuomilehto J, Lindström J, Eriksson JG et al. Prevention of type 2 diabetes mellitus by changes in lifestyle among subjects with impaired glucose tolerance. N Engl J Med 2001; 344: 1343–50.

14. Knowler WC, Barrett-Connor E, Fowler SE et al. Reduction in the incidence of type 2 diabetes with lifestyle intervention or metformin. N Engl J Med 2002; 346: 393–403.

15. Stefanick ML, Mackey S, Sheehan M, Ellsworth N, Haskall WL, Wood PD. Effects of diet and exercise in men and postmenopausal women with low levels of HDL cholesterol and high levels of LDL cholesterol. N Engl J Med 1998; 339:12–20.

16. United Kingdom prospective diabetes study group. Tight blood pressure control and risk of macrovascular and microvascular complications in type 2 diabetes. UKPDS 38. Br Med J 1998; 317: 703–13.

17. Rose G. The Strategy of Preventive Medicine. Oxford: Oxford University Press, 1992.

Chapter 5

How far should BPs be lowered?

Prospective observational data suggest that the lower the blood pressure (BP) the lower the risk of adverse cardiovascular outcomes (see Fig. 1.2). Nevertheless some observational and trial evidence have been reported to suggest that there may be a J-shaped relationship with BP whereby the lowest levels of BP may be associated with increased cardiovascular morbidity or mortality. This largely appears to be due to a misinterpretation of the data, brought about by 'reversed causation', that is, that in certain circumstances, low BP is the result rather than the cause of a pathological condition (for example heart failure) that is linked to increased risk of morbidity and mortality. Similarly chronic vascular damage in the capitance vessels associated with raised arterial pressure is associated with falling diastolic BP in elderly subjects. Hence it is not surprising that short-term follow-up of those with the lowest levels of particularly diastolic BP will be associated with increased cardiovascular risk.

The critical clinical question of how far BP should be lowered remains unanswered by randomised, controlled trial (RCT) data. However, best evidence to date has failed to demonstrate a target below which there is an apparent downside to lowering BP in terms of major cardiovascular events.

Particular concerns have been raised in relation to BP lowering in those with established coronary disease, those with left ventricular hypertrophy (LVH) or post-stroke and, as described in Chapter 6, p. 65, these concerns have not been found to be justified in large morbidity/mortality trials. Furthermore, in the Systolic Hypertension in the Elderly Program (SHEP) trial of the management of isolated systolic hypertension in the elderly,[1] the diastolic BP fell to 68 mmHg in the actively treated group – a reduction that was associated with a significant reduction in cardiovascular events. Further reassurance regarding effective BP lowering arises from the many heart failure trials in which BP tends to start low and the use of drugs that lower BP whilst treating heart failure, (typically diuretics and angiotensin II receptor blockers (ARBs) or angiotensin-converting enzyme (ACE) inhibitors) produced significant reductions in coronary events and death.[2] In short, concerns about 'overtreatment' and a 'J-effect' appear to be largely misplaced.

To date the four trials designed to evaluate how far BP should be lowered are the Hypertensin Optimal Treatment (HOT),[3] UK Prospective Diabetes Study Group (UKPDS),[4] ABCD–NT,[5] and ABCD-H-T[6] trials. However the latter three trials relate only to patients with diabetes. In overview the results of these trials support a 'lower the better' approach.[7]

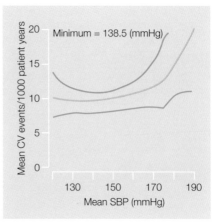

Fig. 5.1 Estimated incidence (95% CI) of CV events by achieved mean SBP.

However, the results of the HOT trial, which have influenced recommendations on target BPs, produced less than robust evidence. This trial was designed to compare the effects of reaching three diastolic targets: ≤ 90, ≤ 85 and ≤ 80 mmHg. Unfortunately the BP range achieved was only 4 mmHg instead of the 10 mmHg required by design. In addition, fewer than expected events occurred. Hence the study was underpowered to evaluate the original question using an intention-to-treat analysis. Consequently, using a less than ideal analysis of achieved BP effects, an optimal pressure of 139/83 mHg was reported.[3] From the data as published however, little advantage was apparent for lowering BP beyond 150/90 mmHg (Fig. 5.1). By contrast, in the diabetic sub-group of the HOT trial, intention-to-treat analyses did confirm large significant reductions in total cardiovascular events in those randomised to reach ≤ 80 mmHg compared with those randomised to ≤ 90 mmHg, even though the actual achieved diastolic and systolic difference was about 4 mmHg (Fig. 5.2).

Further sub-group analyses, which require cautious interpretation, suggest that among various subgroups of non-smokers, the lowest BP strata did enjoy significantly lower event rates.[8]

The data from UKPDS and the two ABCD trials support the results found among patients with diabetes in the HOT trial – that further BP lowering is advantageous. However evidence for lowering systolic BP below

140 mmHg in these trials are not compelling.

The results of the PROGRESS,[9] Heart Outcomes Prevention Evaluation (HOPE),[10] and European trial On Reduction of cardiac events with Perindopril in Stable coronary Artery disease (EUROPA)[11] trials reaffirmed benefits of additional BP lowering irrespective of baseline BP levels among patients with established vascular disease. Hence the targets suggested by the HOT trial are likely to be too high in such high-risk patients. Finally some of

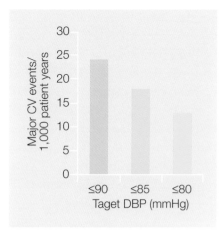

Fig. 5.2 Significant benefits from intensive blood pressure reduction in diabetes (HOT trial).

the benefits observed in the ALLHAT trial[12] (see Ch. 6, p. 70) of a diuretic over both an ACE inhibitor and an alpha-blocker probably result from the better BP lowering achieved in the diuretic group. These benefits observed in ALLHAT were achieved in relation to mean systolic BP levels of 134 mmHg, compared with 136 mmHg.

A summary of currently recommended targets in recent guidelines is shown in Table 5.1, although in summary it seems reasonable to believe that lower values than those recommensed are probably beneficial if tolerated.

JNC 7	ESH-ESC	WHO-ISH	BHS 2004
<140/90 mmHg	<140/90 mmHg	SBP <140 mmHg	<140/85 mmHg
DM renal <130/80	lower if tolerated DM <130/80	DM renal CVD <130/80	DM <130/80

DM: type 2 diabetes CVD: cardiovascular disease Renal: Renal impairment.

Table 5.1 BP targets in various recent guidelines.

Summary

- Robust trial evidence for optimal BP targets does not exist and should be produced.

- Meanwhile current British Hypertension Society targets are recommended (see Table 5.1).

- Targets should be lower for those with diabetes or those with established vascular disease.

References

1. SHEP Collaborative Research Group. Prevention of stroke by antihypertensive drug treatment in older persons with isolated systolic hypertension: final results of the Systolic Hypertension in the Elderly Program (SHEP). JAMA 1991; 265: 3255–64.

2. Garg R, Yusuf S. Overview of randomized trials of angiotensin-converting enzyme inhibitors on mortality and morbidity in patients with heart failure. Collaborative Group on ACE Inhibitor Trials. JAMA 1995; 273: 1450–6.

3. Hansson L, Zanchetti A, Carruthers SG *et al.* Effects of intensive blood-pressure lowering and low-dose aspirin in patients with hypertension: principal results of the Hypertension Optimal Treatment (HOT) randomised trial. *Lancet* 1998; **351**: 1755–62.

4. UK Prospective Diabetes Study Group. Tight blood pressure control and risk of macrovascular and microvascular complications in Type 2 diabetes. UKPDS38. *Br Med J* 1998; **317**: 703–13.

5. Schrier RW, Estacio RO, Esler A, Mehler P. Effects of aggressive blood pressure control in normotensive type 2 diabetic patients on albuminuria, retinopathy and stroke. *Kidney Int* 2002; **61**: 1086–97.

6. Estacio RO, Jeffers BW, Hiatt WR, Biggerstaff SL, Gifford N, Schrier RW. The effect of nisoldipine as compared with enalapril on cardiovascular outcomes in patients with non-insulin independent diabetes and hypertension. *N Engl J Med* 1998; **338**: 645–52.

7. Blood Pressure Lowering Treatment Trialists' Collaboration. Effects of ACE inhibitors, calcium antagonists, and other blood-pressure-lowering drugs: results of prospectively designed overviews of randomised trials. *Lancet* 2000; **356**: 1955–64.

8. Zanchetti A, Hansson L, Clement D *et al* on behalf of the HOT Study Group. Benefits and risks of more intensive blood pressure lowering in hypertensive patients of the HOT Study with different risk profiles: does a J-shaped curve exist in smokers? *J Hypertens* 2003; **21**: 797–804.

9. PROGRESS Collaborative Study Group. Randomised trial of perindopril based blood pressure-lowering regimen among 6108 individuals with previous stroke or transient ischaemic attack. *Lancet* 2001; **358**: 1033–41.

10. The Heart Outcomes Prevention Evaluation Study Investigators. Effects of an angiotensin-converting-enzyme inhibitor, ramipril, on cardiovascular events in high-risk patients. *N Engl J Med* 2000; **342**: 145–53.

11. The EURopean trial On reduction of cardiac events with Perindopril in stable coronary Artery disease investigators. Efficacy of perindopril in reduction of cardiovascular events among patients with stable coronary artery disease: randomised, double-blind, placebo-controlled, multicentre trial (the EUROPA study). Lancet 2003; 362: 782–8.

12. The ALLHAT Officers and Coordinators for the ALLHAT Collaborative Research Group. Major outcomes in high-risk hypertensive patients randomized to angiotensin-converting enzyme inhibitor or calcium channel blocker vs diuretic: The Antihypertensive and Lipid-Lowering treatment to prevent Heart Attack Trial (ALLHAT). *JAMA* 2002; **288**: 2981–97.

Chapter 6

Drug treatment

Trial evidence as of 1993/94

The introduction of antihypertensive drug therapy revolutionised the fate of patients with malignant hypertension for whom death had been an almost inevitable and rapid outcome.[1] Thereafter trials of severe and moderate hypertension confirmed the protective benefits of blood pressure (BP) lowering. Subsequently, during the 1970s,1980s and early 1990s a series of placebo-controlled trials of milder levels of hypertension were carried out.

When the results of these intervention trials with older drug regimens were pooled in 1990,[2] treatment was found to have reduced the risk of stroke by about 38% and that of non-fatal myocardial infarction (MI) and coronary heart disease (CHD) death by about 16% (Fig. 6.1). The impact on coronary events represented an apparent shortfall in benefit expected from prospective observational data.[3] The effects on stroke events were however what was predicted from prospective observational data.[3]

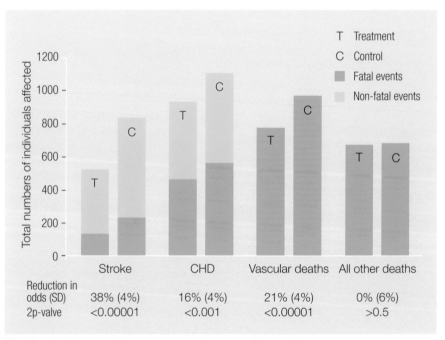

Fig. 6.1 Antihypertensive treatment reduces cardiovascular events.

Despite the benefit of having 17 major morbidity/mortality trials to guide practice, several key unresolved issues in the treatment of hypertension remained. These included:

1. At what level should BP therapy be initiated (i.e optimal thresholds, see Ch. 3, p. 44) and to what level should BP be lowered (i.e. targets, see Ch. 5, p. 62)?

2. Would other concomitant medications (e.g. lipid-lowering or aspirin) provide further benefits? (see Ch. 7, p. 96).

3. Would treatment with more contemporary drugs such as calcium channel blockers (CCBs), alpha-blockers, angiotensin-converting enzyme (ACE) inhibitors, and angiotensin receptor blockers (ARBs) result in greater protection against CHD events compared with diuretics or beta-blockers with which there appeared to have been a shortfall in trials hitherto?

4. Would specific combinations of antihypertensive agents confer benefits over other combinations?

5. To what extent would the answers to these questions vary in specific sub-groups of patients?

This chapter will attempt to address the last three questions:

Benefits of more contemporary drugs over standard therapy

Systolic Hypertension in Europe Trial (SYST-EUR)[4]

This was the first prospective, randomised, placebo-controlled trial to evaluate the effect of a drug class other than a diuretic or beta-blocker – in this case a dihydropyridine CCB – as first-line antihypertensive treatment. It was the second trial after SHEP[5] designed to evaluate whether drug treatment of isolated systolic hypertension (ISH) would improve cardiovascular outcomes. During the conduct of this trial of 4695 patients, the results of the SHEP trial showed that major cardiovascular benefits accrued from the treatment of ISH, with a diuretic-based regimen. The results of SHEP were supportive of those arising from sub-group analyses of ISH patients in the MRC trial of the treatment of older patients.[6]

Despite these earlier results, the SYST-EUR trial continued and thereby allowed the important question as to whether the diuretic-based benefits seen in SHEP and the MRC trial could be attained using the CCB nitrendipine. SYST-EUR was stopped early because of unequivocal benefits of the CCB-based treatment on the primary end-point of stroke. The magnitude of the benefit – a 42% reduction – was at least as large as had been achieved with diuretics in earlier trials.

Captopril Primary Prevention Trial (CAPPP)[7]

This trial was designed to be the first study to compare the benefits of a 'newer' agent (the ACE inhibitor captopril) with one of the standard first-line agents – in this case a beta-blocker. The trial included 10,985 hypertensive patients and the primary outcome of cardiovascular morbidity and mortality was not differentially influenced by the two treatment regimens, although a number of secondary end-points were differentially affected, e.g. stroke incidence was higher in those randomised to captopril. However the results of this study should be interpreted with great caution because it was seriously flawed in two respects.

Firstly, despite randomisation, the two groups were markedly unbalanced at baseline. For example there were more diabetic patients in those randomised to captopril. It is thought that this came about because the randomisation process involved sealed envelopes, which gave the investigator the opportunity to influence the allocation of treatment to patients.

The second major problem with CAPPP was that the BP levels were substantially higher throughout the trial in those randomised to the ACE inhibitor because up to two-thirds of the patients in the captopril group were given the drug once daily, rather than the ideal of three times daily if optimal 24-hour BP reduction is to be achieved. This study therefore did not contribute to evaluating whether newer drugs, specifically an ACE inhibitor, confers additional cardiovascular protection over conventional therapy.

It is surprising and important to note that although several ACE inhibitor-based trials have shown convincing benefits in the treatment of heart failure and left ventricular dysfunction,[8] and other studies suggest treatment benefits in sub-groups of patients with renal disease and type 1 diabetes,[9] there have been no placebo-controlled trials of ACE inhibitors in hypertension.

Swedish Trial in Older Patients with Hypertension-2 (STOP-2)[10]

STOP-2 included 6414 patients followed up for an average of 5 years, and like CAPPP, it was designed to compare conventional drug treatment (thiazide ± beta-blocker) with newer treatments, in this case either a CCB-based or ACE inhibitor-based regimen. The design of this trial, like CAPPP, was powered on the basis that newer treatments would reduce cardiovascular morbidity and mortality by 25% compared with older drugs. This was unrealistic given that based on the meta-analysis of trials up to that time, any benefits of newer agents were only likely to accrue in relation to coronary rather than stroke events. Predictably perhaps, there were no significant differences in total cardiovascular events in those receiving newer drugs or conventional drugs. These results were further complicated by crossover of drugs used as add-on therapy among the three comparator groups.

International Nifedipine GITS Study: intervention as a Goal in Hypertension Treatment (INSIGHT)[11]

INSIGHT was designed to test the primary hypothesis that a dihydropyridine CCB (nifedipine GITS) would reduce the combined cardiovascular end-points of cardiovascular death, MI, heart failure and stroke by 25% (once again an unlikely difference) compared with a hydrochlorothiazide/amiloride combination-based treatment regimen. Atenolol was a common add-on therapy to both limbs of the study, if required.

A total of 6321 hypertensive patients, with at least one additional cardiovascular risk factor, were randomised and followed up for a median period of approximately 3.5 years. BP levels were lowered equally well in the two groups and there were no significant differences in the incidence of primary or secondary end-points in the two treatment groups.

Nordic Diltiazem Study (NORDIL)[12]

NORDIL was similar to INSIGHT in that it compared a CCB (albeit the non-dihydropyridine, diltiazem) with a reference regimen of either diuretic or beta-blocker. The study included 10,916 patients and was powered to detect a 20% relative risk reduction in combined cardiovascular events.

After an average follow-up period of 4.5 years, the incidence of primary end-points in the two limbs of the trial was almost identical. Interestingly, significantly fewer strokes occurred in the diltiazem arm (a 20% reduction) despite smaller falls in BP in the diltazem group.

Antihypertensive and Lipid-Lowering treatment to prevent a Heart Attack Trial (ALLHAT)[13]

This is, to date, the largest hypertension trial to have been conducted. It was unique in attempting to address which of four first-line agents was best able to prevent CHD events in hypertensive subjects. An outline of the design of ALLHAT is shown in Figure 6.2. Initially, over 40,000 patients were randomised, double-blind, to receive either the CCB, amlodipine, ACE inhibitor lisinopril, alpha-blocker doxazosin, or the primary comparator – diuretic chlorthalidone. In a sub-group of over 10,000 of these patients, the effects of the cholesterol-lowering drug, pravastatin, were compared with usual care (see Chap 7, p. 97). The study was planned for an average follow-up period of 6 years.

After a mean follow-up period of about 3 years, the alpha-blocker limb of the trial was stopped early on the grounds that there was an apparent excess of cardiovascular events (mainly heart failure) in those allocated to the alpha-blocker, compared with the diuretic.[14] No outcome differences were observed between the two groups in the primary end-point, fatal CHD and non-fatal MI, nor in all-cause mortality despite

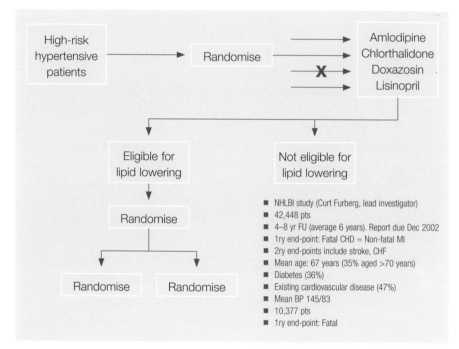

Fig. 6.2 Summary of ALLHAT.

significantly less BP reduction (3 mmHg systolic) achieved in the alpha-blocker limb. Interpretation of the apparent increase in heart failure associated with doxazosin is controversial.[15] Whatever the explanation, it is a great shame that the premature termination of this limb of the trial has resulted in the relegation of this drug to a remote add-on role in BP management.

For the remainder of the trial, following an average intervention period of about 5 years, the primary outcome of combined fatal CHD or non-fatal MI was not significantly different between the remaining three treatment arms of the study. In the ALLHAT population, which consisted of 47% women and 32% African-Americans, the ACE inhibitor lisinopril was significantly less effective at lowering BP than either the diuretic or the CCB. The differences in secondary end-points, notably stroke incidence (significantly higher among those on the ACE inhibitor compared with the diuretic-treated group) could be explained by the relative lack of efficacy on BP reduction with the ACE inhibitor compared with the other drugs. The most striking and controversial finding in ALLHAT was an apparent excess of congestive heart failure seen both with the CCB (increased by 38% compared with a diuretic) and the ACE inhibitor (increased by 20% compared with a diuretic). However, the lack of any increased mortality associated with the increased heart failure, raises the question, as it did in the case of the alpha-blocker limb, as to whether this largely non-validated end-point was indeed heart failure in the strict sense of the definition. Recruitment into ALLHAT necessitated the withdrawal of previous therapies that would have included diuretics in many patients. Such withdrawal could lead to fluid retention, thereby unmasking previously treated or pre-empted heart failure and lead to an apparent excess of heart failure in those patients not allocated to chlorthalidone. The diagnosis of heart failure may have been further complicated or confused by the side effect of pedal oedema, which is frequently induced by the CCB and, to a lesser extent, doxazosin.

One clear piece of evidence from ALLHAT was that there was no excess of coronary events associated with the CCB and this important finding from a randomised, controlled study highlights serious flaws in the interpretation of earlier uncontrolled observational studies suggesting that not only were CCBs associated with increased coronary risk, but also with other non-cardiovascular events.[16]

An advantage of ALLHAT is that by virtue of its design and study size, meaningful analyses of sub-groups of patients such as diabetics, African-Americans and females were undertaken (Tables 6.1 and 6.2). Clearly African-Americans were disadvantaged by ACE inhibitor-based treatment compared with diuretics, presumably reflecting the lack of efficacy of the ACE inhibitor on BP control, which was particularly apparent in this ethnic group. Perhaps more surprisingly, ALLHAT did not confirm significant advantages of any of the treatment limbs, notably ACE inhibitors, compared with chlorthalidone in the sub-group of patients with diabetes.

The extrapolation of ALLHAT data to more contemporary treatment regimens is problematic in many respects. The diuretic used in ALLHAT, chlorthalidone, is rarely used outside north America and it is questionable as to whether the nature of the drug and the average doses used in ALLHAT are equivalent to 'low-dose thiazides' such

	1° end-point	Total mortality	Stroke	Comb CHD	Comb CVD	CHF
Total	–	–	–	–	–	a
< 65 years	–	–	–	–	–	a
≥ 65 years	–	–	–	–	–	a
Men	–	–	–	–	–	a
Women	–	–	–	–	–	a
Black	–	–	–	–	–	a
Non-black	–	–	–	–	–	a
Diabetic	–	–	–	–	–	a
Non-diabetic	–	–	–	–	–	a

– No significant differance between drug groups.
a Significant outcome in favour of chlorthalidone
CHD Coronary heart disease CVD cardiovascular disease CHF Congestive heart failure

Table. 6.1 ALLHAT trial results. Sub-groups: Amlodipine vs chlorthalidone.

	1° end-point	Tot mortality	Stroke	Comb CHD	Comb CVD	CHF
Total	–	–	a	–	a	a
< 65 years	–	–	–	–	–	a
≥ 65 years	–	–	–	a	a	a
Men	–	–	–	–	a	a
Women	–	–	a	–	a	a
Black	–	–	a	a	a	a
Non-black	–	–	–	–	–	a
Diabetic	–	–	–	–	–	a
Non-diabetic	–	–	a	–	a	a

– No significant differance between drug groups.
a Significant outcome in favour of chlorthalidone
CHD Coronary heart disease CVD cardiovascular disease CHF Congestive heart failure

Table. 6.2 ALLHAT trial results. Sub-groups: Lisinopril vs chlorthalidone.

as bendrofluazide (2mg) or hydrochlorothiazide (12.5mg), which are currently recommended in many parts of the world. There are important pharmacological differences between chlorthalidone and thiazides, and the significant hypokalaemia observed and treated in many patients receiving chlorthalidone in ALLHAT raises the question of dose equivalence to more usual low-dose thiazide treatments.

In addition, most patients needed at least two drugs to reach the BP targets stipulated in the trial and in order to avoid crossover treatments affecting the first-line drug comparisons, a number of largely obsolete add-on drugs such as reserpine, clonidine, and hydralazine were incorporated into the treatment strategies. The idea of blanket superiority of 'thiazide-like diuretics' over the CCB used in ALLHAT – a conclusion that has arisen from the trial – does not appear commensurate with the actual data.

Second Australian National Blood Pressure Study (ANBP2)[17]

This trial of 6083 patients aged 65–84 was designed to compare the effects of an ACE inhibitor-based regimen (usually enalapril) with those of a thiazide-based regimen (usually hydrochlorothiazide). This trial is almost unique in that it did actually include a truly low dose of thiazide (12.5 mg). The results suggested that those allocated to ACE inhibition had a non-significant reduction in the primary end-point of death or total cardiovascular events. Interestingly, these benefits were peculiar to men and interpretation was further complicated by the fact that compliance was only about 60% with a minority (38%) taking monotherapy. These data appear to conflict with the ALLHAT results and generally appear to be less reliable.

The obvious deficiencies of many of these recently reported trials comparing 'new' and 'older' therapies was that they lacked the power to detect differences in CHD outcome which, based on earlier meta-analysis, was the source of a shortfall in benefit. A realistic hypothesis might be that newer drugs would confer greater protection against CHD, and several studies (not designed in hypertensive subjects) provide credence for this idea. In order to test this hypothesis, two courses of action have been followed. The first demanded studies with adequate numbers of patients randomized to detect a 20% relative risk reduction in CHD end-points between treatment groups. Two studies were powered to address this critical question: ALLHAT as detailed earlier,[13] and the Anglo-Scandinavian Cardiac Outcomes Trial (ASCOT)[18] which is described later in this chapter. The second course of action was to conduct further pooled analyses of available trial data.

Meta-analyses

In 2000, the Blood Pressure Lowering Treatment Trialists (BPLT) Collaboration published the first of these meta-analyses, which represented an overview of data from 15 trials and approximately 75,000 patients.[19] It is important to emphasize that all eligible trials had to conform to pre-specified criteria and the collaborators agreed to a programme of prospectively designed overviews.

The main conclusions from these important analyses (Figure 6.3) is that, based on the trials included before the year 2000, overall cardiovascular events are not differentially influenced by different treatment regimens based on older or newer drugs. Nevertheless, the total number of patients whose data have been analysed were still too few to allow definitive conclusions to be made about the lack of benefits of any particular treatment regimen and no analyses have been undertaken on particular patient sub-groups. This analysis has, however, shown certain trends of differences, for example stroke events appeared to be somewhat lower, and CHD events including heart failure somewhat higher with CCB regimens than with older drugs. In the case of ACE inhibitors, no significant differences have been observed compared with diuretic or beta-blocker-based regimens, except for the expected trend in favour of ACE inhibitors in the case of heart failure.

As the authors of this overview emphasize, substantial new information has been provided, but many questions remain unanswered. The most recent meta-analyses from the Blood Pressure Lowering Trialists Collaboration and others provide an update of all currently available trial evidence, including ALLHAT,[13] ANBP2,[17] LIFE,[20] and SCOPE.[21] The findings are

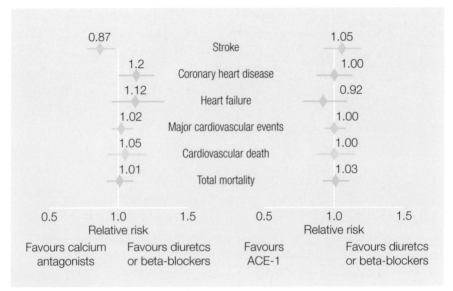

Fig. 6.3 WHO-ISH meta-analysis.[19]

consistent with those of the BPLT in 2000, in that the main source of benefit from BP-lowering drugs appears to be due to BP lowering itself and there is little evidence of additional class-specific benefits over and above the BP lowering effect they produce. The only possible exceptions to this general comment are:

- CCBs appear to be less protective against heart failure than other classes of agents.
- Compelling indications for certain drugs do exist (see Table 6.2).
- ARB drugs may provide extra stroke protection.
- Newer drugs appear to produce less new-onset diabetes than older drugs (especially when diuretics and beta-blockers are combined).

Choosing the first-line agent

The heterogeneity of hypertensive patients accounts for varying and often unpredictable BP responses to individual hypertensive drugs[22]

Class	Condition favouring the use	Compelling	Possible
Diuretics (thiazides)	Congestive heart failure; elderly hypertensives; isolated systolic hypertension; hypertensives of African origin	Gout	Pregnancy
Diuretics (loop)	Renal insufficiency; congestive heart failure		
Diuretcis (anti-aldosterone)	Congestive heart failure; post-myocardial infarction	Renal failure; hyperkalaemia	
Beta-blockers	Angina pectoris; post-myocardial infarction; congestive heart failure (up-titration); pregnancy; tachyarrhythmias	Asthma; chronic obstructive pulmonary disease; A-V block (grade 2 or 3)	Peripheral vascular disease; glucose intolerance; athletes and physically active patients
Calcium antagonists (dihydropyridines)	Elderly patients; isolated systolic hypertension; angina pectoris; peripheral vascular disease; carotid atherosclerosis; pregnancy		Tachyarrhythmias; congestive heart failure
Calcium antagonists (verapamil, diltiazem)	Angina pectoris; carotid atherosclerosis; supraventricular tachycardia	A-V block (grade 2 or 3); congestive heart failure	
Angiotensin-converting enzyme (ACE) inhibitors	Congestive heart failure; LV dysfunction; post-myocardial infarction; type 1 diabetic nephropathy; proteinuria	Pregnancy; hyperkalaemia; bilateral renal artery stenosis	
Angiotensin II receptor antagonists (AT$_1$-blockers)	Type 2 diabetic nephropathy; diabetic microalbuminuria; proteinuria; left ventricular hypertrophy; ACE-inhibitor cough	Pregnancy; hyperkalaemia; bilateral renal artery stenosis	
Alpha-blockers	Prostatic hyperplasia (BPH); hyperlipidaemia	Orthostatic hypotension	Congestive heart failure

A-V, atrioventricular; LV, left ventricular

Table 6.3a Summary of ALLHAT.

and with one or two exceptions,[23] no distinct patient phenotypes dictate that choice of individual drugs. This means that for many patients drug selection is based on trial and error.

In general, the BP of older patients and those of African origin tend to respond better to diuretics and CCB drugs, whereas younger Caucasian patients respond better to beta-blockers and either ACE inhibitors or ARBs than to diuretics or CCBs.[23,24] It must be emphasised that these are broad generalisations and there are many exceptions to the rule.

For each major class of antihypertensive drug there are compelling indications and contraindications for their use in particular patient groups, based on trial experience (Table 6.3a and b). In other instances recommendations may be made, based upon evidence that is less robust.

In the absence of special considerations, cost is an important issue, and the least expensive agent – which is a low-dose diuretic in most countries – should be used, particularly since this class of agent is a good companion with most other drug classes.

Dose titration is recommended, where necessary, to achieve goal BPs, for all drugs except diuretics, but this approach may be limited by the appearance of side effects. This may be avoided by either dose reduction and combination therapy, or a switch to an alternative agent.

What is the optimal pair of BP-lowering agents?

Evidence from several trials[26,27] show that the majority of patients with hypertension require at least two BP-lowering agents if currently recommended targets are to be reached (Fig. 6.4).

Whilst the vast majority of trials of BP management have involved the use of BP-lowering regimens including two or more agents, the choice of a second or third agent has usually been unstructured. Hence the results of these trials cannot inform recommendations for optimal combinations of anti-hypertensive agents. Advice is therefore based on the theoretical benefits of selecting agents that have complimentary rather than overlapping mechanisms of action. This has given rise to several similar recommendations

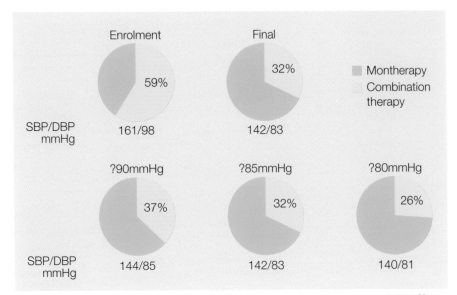

Fig. 6.4 Combination therapy needed to achieve target blood pressures (HOT).[26]

as shown in Figure 6.5. More recently the ESH–ESC guidelines have produced a further version of these earlier models (Fig. 6.6).

This latest European version contradicts earlier versions in that CCBs and diuretics are considered a logical combination despite sharing, at

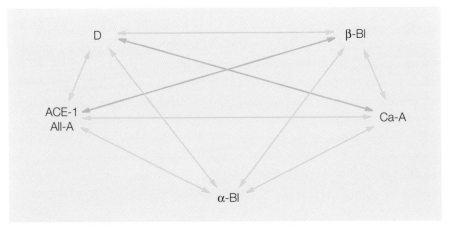

Fig. 6.5 Combination therapy needed to achieve target blood pressure.

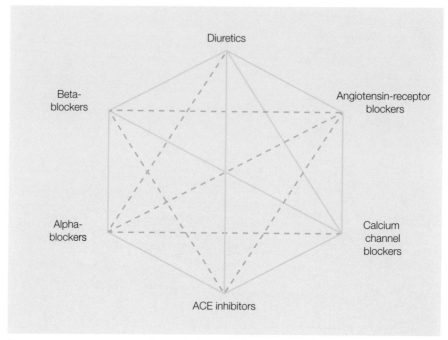

Fig. 6.6 Possible combinations of different classes of antihypertensive agents. The most rational combinations are represented as thick lines. The frames indicated classes of antihypertensive agents proven to be beneficial in controlled interventional trials.[25]

least in part, the common mechanism of action. Furthermore these two agents have in earlier studies been shown not to produce optimal BP lowering when used in combination.[28] Interestingly as shown in Table 6.4 this combination – logical or not – is in common use, at least in the UK.[29] A further change in the European 'star' compared with earlier recommendations is the suggestion that alpha-blockers should not be used in combination with any other agents except beta-blockers. This may well have been driven by the results of ALLHAT[14] (see Ch. 6, p. 70) but evidence on drug combinations cannot be drawn from ALLHAT due to the trial design and, from a mechanistic viewpoint, this group of agents should be complimentary with all other drug classes.

The British Hypertension Society (BHS) have recently published a proposed algorithm – the ABCD approach – for how best to combine

Drugs	1994 (%)	1998 (%)
Diuretic + ß-blocker	41±2.45	21±1.93
Diuretic + calcium antagonist	19±1.96	21±1.93
Diuretic + ACE inhibitor	15±1.78	27±2.1
Other	25±2.16	31±2.2

Table. 6.4 Type of drug used by those receiving 2 drugs for hypertension, 1994–98.

drugs to achieve optimal BP control[30] (see Fig. 6.7). Each letter refers to a BP-lowering drug class: (A = ACE inhibitor or ARB; B = beta-blocker; C = dihydropyridine CCB; D = diuretic) and the theory underpinning this approach is that hypertension can be broadly classified as 'high renin' or

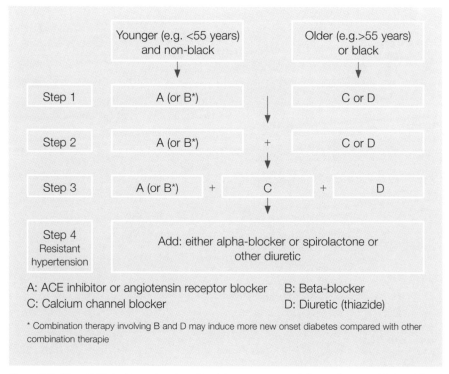

Fig. 6.7 The British Hypertension Society recommendations for combining blood pressure lowering drugs.

'low renin'. The former is therefore best treated by those classes which inhibit the renin–angiotensin system (A or B), and the latter by those classes that do not (C or D).[23,24]

In general, younger people (< 55 years) and Caucasians tend to have higher renin status than older people (≥ 55 years) or black people, hence the recommended allocation of drugs for step 1 based on age and race shown in Figure 6.7. The rationale for steps 2, 3 and 4 are less soundly based, and are recommended on the logical grounds of selecting combinations of agents which do not have overlapping mechanisms.

Finally the ABCD treatment algorithm has the added advantage of providing advice on how best to control more severe levels of raised BP. For those patients with apparently resistant hypertension despite taking several conventional agents, the use of aldosterone antagonists (e.g. spironolactone 25 mg o.d.) appears to provide (albeit on an anecdotal level) dramatic BP-lowering effects.

The BHS,[31] JNC 7,[32] and European guidance[25] have all moved towards recommending the use of fixed low-dose combinations of drugs. Historically the use of such agents has been considered infra dig, but in light of the real need for more than one agent for most patients[26,27] and the fact that doctors do not tend to titrate therapy, it seems a logical approach that should enhance compliance and BP lowering. With this in mind the BHS, JNC7 and the latest European guidelines formally recommend combination therapy as first-line treatment (see Figs 3.2 and 6.8).

Despite the need to use two or more drugs for BP control in most patients, ASCOT is the only trial specifically designed to compare the effects of different combinations of antihypertensive treatment[18] as shown in Figure 6.9. This trial compares the effect of the standard regimen (beta-blocker +/– diuretic) with a newer regimen (CCB +/– ACE-inhibitor) in over 19,000 patients with hypertension. A common add-on drug of doxazosin GITS is used for both limbs if BP targets are not reached. The primary end-point is non-fatal myocardial infarction and fatal CHD, and the trial is due to report in 2005.

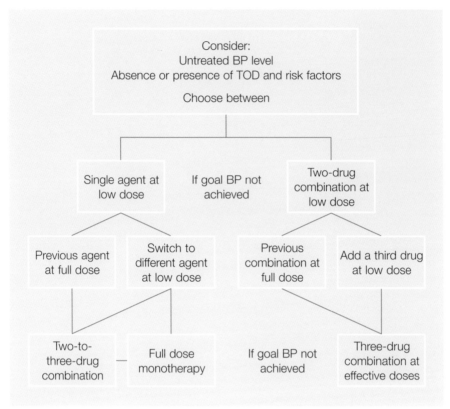

Fig. 6.8 ESH-ESC use of monotherapy or combination therapy.[25]

Which drugs are best for different sub-groups of patients?

Diabetes

Cardiovascular morbidity and mortality rates are high in patients with hypertension and diabetes. Higher BP levels are instrumental in the pathophysiology of macrovascular and microvascular disease and the potential benefits of therapeutic intervention on BP are therefore large. Although several studies have included significant subgroups of diabetic patients, only one major trial of BP lowering powered to evaluate major cardiovascular end-points specifically in patients with type 2 diabetes has been carried out to date – the United

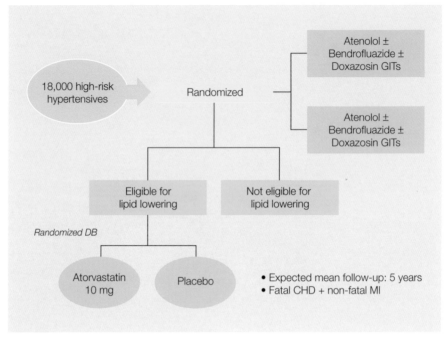

Fig. 6.9 ASCOT probe design.

Kingdom Prospective Diabetes Study – UKPDS.[27] This long-awaited study included a BP-lowering limb which evaluated macrovascular and microvascular end-points as a function of different degrees of BP lowering in 1148 hypertensive patients with type 2 diabetes. There were unequivocal benefits associated with tight compared with less tight BP control in terms of any diabetes-related end-point (34%) and macrovascular outcomes (stroke reduction 44%, CHD reduction 31%). These benefits were markedly greater than those associated with greater or lesser improvements in HbA1C, which did not impact significantly on macrovascular events, although benefits on CHD events were of borderline significance.

These findings were supported by the sub-group analysis of the diabetic patients in the diabetic patients in the HOT study (see Fig. 5.2) and provide good support for the recommendations to lower target BPs in patients with type 2 diabetes.

The attempt to compare outcomes in the two BP treatment groups in this part of the UKPDS trial – one ACE inhibitor based (captopril) and one beta-blocker based (atenolol) – requires very careful interpretation.[27] This randomised comparison of only 758 patients provided no evidence of any difference in cardiovascular event rates between the two groups. However this aspect of the study had negligible power to detect potentially important differences between the two groups. Nevertheless, the apparent 'equivalence' of treatment has been accepted both by many diabetologists and other practitioners, despite the obvious potential for a type 2 statistical error.

The largest sub-group of diabetic patients studied in a hypertension trial was that included in ALLHAT.[13] In contradiction of a belief strongly held by many physicians, those allocated to ACE inhibitors did not gain any benefits in terms of cardiovascular disease (CVD) prevention compared with those on diretics, and those on CCBs did equally well as those on diuretics or ACE inhibitors (see Tables 6.1 and 6.2).

Three studies have shown that ARBs provide a renoprotective effect and reduce renal morbidity in type 2 diabetic patients with nephropathy.[33,34,35] These effects appear to be independent of BP reduction.

Study of the Effects of Irbesartan on Microalbuminuria in Hypertensive Patients with Type 2 Diabetes (IRMA2)[33]

In this trial 590 hypertensive patients with type 2 diabetes and microalbuminuria were randomised to either irbesartan (150–300 mg daily) or placebo, added to usual antihypertensive therapy (excluding ACE inhibitors). The primary outcome, of progression to overt proteinuria or a 30% increase in urinary albumin excretion rate, was significantly reduced by 70% in the group treated with irbesartan 300 mg and by 30% in those treated with irbesartan150 mg.

Reduction of End-points in Non-insulin Dependent Diabetes Mellitus with the Angiotensin 2 Antagonist Losartan (RENAAL)[34]

In this trial, 1513 patients with type 2 diabetes, proteinuria and raised serum creatinine, were randomised to either losartan (maximum dose 100 mg) or placebo in addition to other antihypertensive drugs. The primary outcome was a composite end-point of doubling of serum creatinine, end-stage renal failure or death, which was significantly reduced by 16% in those randomised to losartan.

Irbesartan Type-2 Diabetic Nephropathy Trial (IDNT)[35]

In this trial, 1715 patients were randomised to receive either irbesartan (maximum dose 300 mg), amlodipine (maximum dose 10 mg) or placebo (other antihypertensive drugs). The primary end-point was the same as in the RENAAL trial. For similar falls in BP in the two pre-specified active treatment groups of 140/77 mmHg and 141/77 mmHg respectively, there was a significant, 23% relative risk reduction in the primary end-point in those randomised to irbesartan compared with the amlodipine group, and a 20% reduction compared with placebo. Importantly, these benefits were not reflected in terms of fewer cardiovascular events (which were secondary end-points) in the irbesartan group compared with either the amlodipine or placebo group.

This highlights the importance, when interpreting trials in high-risk patients, of effects on major cardiovascular benefits, rather than surrogate end-points before recommendations for the use of particular drug classes can be made.

On this basis of an overview of all BP-lowering trials including patients with type 2 diabetes, and particularly the results of the HOT trial,[26] lower target BPs for this group of patients are recommended.[25,31,32] Furthermore it seems likely that effective BP lowering, rather than the choice of drug, is the critical issue. Nevertheless trial evidence shows that the vast majority of type 2 diabetic patients require at least two antihypertensive agents to control BP[27] and overall best evidence suggests that a drug that blocks the renin–angiotensin system should be part of any such regimen.

Results from the diabetic subgroup in the LIFE trial[36] provide strong evidence to support the use of ARBs in patients with hypertension and diabetes, especially when complicated by left ventricular hypertrophy (LVH).

In patients with type 1 diabetes, treatment regimens based on ACE inhibitors have been claimed to reduce the rate of decline in renal functions,[9] although to what extent these benefits were independent of BP reduction remains controversial.[37]

LVH

Many small, usually inadequately designed trials evaluating the effects of various drug classes on regression of LVH have been published. Meta-analyses of these studies which have been produced[38,39] suggest that ACE inhibitors and CCBs may be more effective at achieving LVH regression than other drug classes. However the implications of these findings, if true, on major cardiovascular events, remains unclear. One trial, the Losartan Intervention For End-point Reduction in Hypertension Study (LIFE)[20] compared the impact of two BP regimens on major cardiovascular events in patients with LVH.

LIFE trial[20]

This trial compared the effects of the ARB losartan (50 mg or 100 mg) with a beta-blocker, atenolol (50 mg or 100 mg) in 9222 patients with essential hypertension and electrocardiogram (ECG)-based LVH. Hydrochlorothiazide was used as a common second-line add-on therapy. Following an average follow-up period of 4 years, BPs were reduced to similar levels by both treatment strategies. The LVH regression was significantly greater in the losartan group than in the atenolol group. There was a statistically significant reduction in the combined primary end-point of cardiovascular death, MI and stroke of 13% in those randomized to losartan compared with those allocated to atenolol. This overall beneficial effect was effectively due to a reduction in strokes, with no benefits in coronary events. Among the sub-group of diabetic subjects, the benefits of losartan were particularly pronounced, with major benefits in all-cause mortality.[36]

This was the first trial to show, for an equivalent degree of BP lowering, a convincing difference in the effect of two drug classes in the primary cardiovascular outcome among hypertensive patients. This implies that treatment effects may be independent of BP lowering. However whether the differential outcome was due to a particular benefit of the ARB or whether, as in the MRC Trial,[6] a beta-blocker regimen is less effective in protection against stroke is unclear.

Other high-risk patients

The possibility of benefits of antihypertensive agents over and above those due to BP lowering was raised in the context of ACE inhibitors as a result of the Heart Outcome Preventive Evaluation (HOPE) trial.[40]

HOPE trial[40]

In this study of 9297 patients at high cardiovascular risk, patients, whether hypertensive or not, were randomised to the ACE inhbitor ramipril, or placebo. Dramatic benefits in all cardiovascular events were reported in association with the use of ramipril, which purportedly only produced a BP-lowering effect of 3/2 mmHg. This small BP reduction was unlikely to explain the major cardiovascular benefits observed. However ramipril was prescribed at night in the HOPE trial and as a relatively short-acting ACE inhibitor, real BP benefits were likely to be underestimated if BPs were measured in a non-standardised way sometime during the day. Indeed in a small substudy of HOPE,[41] ABPM was carried out on 38 subjects. Significant mean daytime BP differences of 10/4 mmHg were observed between those receiving ramipril and those receiving placebo, and significant night-time differences of 17/8 mmHg were also recorded. If such differences were applicable to the whole HOPE population, the cardiovascular benefits attributed to non-related benefits of ramipril are totally explainable by effects on BP.

PROGRESS trial[42]

This study of over 6000 patients who had established cerebrovascular disease (stroke or transcient ischaemic attack) was designed to evaluate whether, irrespective of BP level, BP lowering with an ACE inhibitor-based regimen – usually in association with the diuretic indapamide – would prevent a further stroke. In short, further stroke was reduced by 28% (P = < 0.0001) in association with the perindopril-based regimen. It should be pointed out however that those who received the ACE inhibitor alone derived very little benefit, whereas those who received the combination of ACE inhibitor plus indapamide derived the benefits expected from the degree of BP lowering achieved. One earlier, little known post-stroke study carried out and published in China,[43] which also used indapamide to lower BP, showed secondary stroke reduction benefits compatible with those observed in PROGRESS.

Summary

- Extensive randomised trial data are available to guide practice.

- Meta-analysis suggest effective BP reduction is probably more important than the agent used to do so.

- Most patients require at least two agents to lower BP levels to current targets.

- Few trial data are available to guide the choice of which pair of agents to use.

References

1. Keith NM, Wagener HP, Barker NW. Some different types of essential hypertension: their cause and prognosis. Am J Med Sci 1939; 197: 332–43.

2. Collins R, Peto R, MacMahon S et al. Blood pressure, stroke, and coronary heart disease. Part 2, Short-term reductions in blood pressure: overview of randomised drug trials in their epidemiological context. Lancet 1990; 335: 827–9.

3. MacMahon et al. BP, Stroke and CHD, Part 1. Lancet 1990; 335: 765–774.

4. Staessen, JA, Fagard R, Thijs L et al for the Systolic Hypertension in Europe (Syst-Eur) Trial Investigators. Randomised double-blind comparison of placebo and active treatment for older patients with isolated systolic hypertension. Lancet 1997; 350: 757–64.

5. SHEP Co-operative Research Group. Prevention of stroke by antihypertensive drug treatment in older persons with isolated systolic hypertension. Final results of the Systolic Hypertension in the Elderly Program (SHEP). J Am Med Assoc 1991; 265: 3255–64.

6. MRC Working Party. Medical Research Council trial of treatment of hypertension in older adults: principal results. Br Med J 1992; 304: 405–12.

7. Hansson L, Lindholm LH, Niskanen L et al for the Captopril Prevention Project (CAPPP) study group. Effect of angiotensin-converting-enzyme inhibition compared with conventional therapy on cardiovascular morbidity and mortality in hypertension: the Captopril Prevention Project (CAPPP) randomised trial. Lancet 1999; 353: 611–16.

8. Garg R, Yusuf S. Overview of randomized trials of angiotensin-converting enzyme inhibitors on mortality and morbidity in patients with heart failure. Collaborative Group on ACE Inhibitor Trials. JAMA 1995; 273: 1450–6.

9. Lewis EJ, Hunsicker LG, Bain RP, Rohde RD for the Collaborative Study Group. The effect of angiotensin converting-enzyme inhibition on diabetic nephropathy. N Engl J Med 1993; 329: 1456–1462.

10. Hansson L, Lindholm LH, Ekborn T et al for the STOP-2 Hypertension Study Group. Randomised trial of old and new antihypertensive drugs in elderly patients: cardiovascular mortality and morbidity. The Swedish Trial in Old Patients with Hypertension-2 study. Lancet 1999; 354: 1751–6.

11. Brown MJ, Palmer CR, Castaigne A, de Leeuw PW, Mancia G, Rosenthal T, Ruilope LM. Morbidity and mortality in patients randomised to double-blind treatment with a long-acting-calcium channel blocker of diuretic in the International Nifedipine GITS study: Intervention as a Goal in Hypertension Treatment (INSIGHT). Lancet 2000; 356: 366–72.

12. Hansson L, Hedner T, Lund-Johansen P et al. Randomised trial of the effects of calcium antagonists compared with diuretics and β-blockers on cardiovascular morbidity and mortality in hypertension on the Nordic Diltiazem study NORDIL. Lancet 2000; 356: 359–65.

13. ALLHAT Officers and Coordinators for the ALLHAT Collaborative Research Group. The Antihypertensive and Lipid-Lowering treatment to prevent Heart Attack Trial. Major outcomes in high-risk hypertensive patients randomized to angiotensin-converting enzyme inhibitor or calcium channel blocker vs diuretic: The Antihypertensive and Lipid-Lowering treatment to prevent Heart Attack Trial (ALLHAT). JAMA 2002; 23: 2981–97.

14. The ALLHAT Officers and Co-ordinators for the ALLHAT Collaborative Research Group. Major cardiovascular events in hypertensive patients randomized to Doxazosin vs Chlorthalidone. The Antihypertensive and Lipid-lowering treatment to prevent Heart Attack Trial (ALLHAT). J Am Med Assoc 2000; 283: 1967–75.

15. Poulter NR, Williams B. Doxazosin for the management of hypertension: implications of the findings of the ALLHAT trial. Am J Hypertens 2001; 14: 1170–2.

16. Stanton AV. Calcium channel blockers. The jury is still out on whether they cause heart attacks and suicide. Br Med J 1998; 316: 1471–3.

17. Wing LMH, Reid CM, Ryan P et al for the Second Australian National Blood Pressure Study Group. A comparison of outcomes with angiotensin-converting-enzyme inhibitors and diuretics for hypertension in the elderly. New Engl J Med 2003; 348: 583–92.

18. Sever PS, Dahlof B, Poulter NR et al. Rationale, design, methods, and baseline demography of participants of the Anglo-Scandinavian Cardiac Outcomes Trial. J Hypertens 2002; 19: 1139–47.

19. Blood Pressure Lowering Treatment Trialists' Collaboration: Effects of ACE inhibitors, calcium antagonists, and other blood-pressure-lowering drugs; results of prospectively designed overviews of randomised trials. Lancet 2000; 356: 1955–64.

20. Dahlof B, Devereux RB, Kjeldsen SE et al for the LIFE Study Group. Cardiovascular morbidity and mortality in the Losartan Intervention For Endpoint reduction in hypertension study (LIFE): a randomised trial against atenolol. Lancet 23 Mar 2002;359(9311): 995–1003.

21. Lithell H, Hansson L, Skoog et al for the SCOPE Study Group. The Study on Cognition and Prognosis in the Elderly (SCOPE): principal results of a randomized double-blind intervention trial. J Hypertens 2003; 21: 875–86.

22. Attwood S, Bird R, Burch K et al. Within-patient correlation between the antihypertensive effects of atenolol, lisinopril and nifedipine. J Hypertens 1994; 12: 1053–60.

23. Dickerson JE et al. Optimalisation of antihypertensive treatment by crossover rotation of four major classes. Lancet 1999; 353: 2008–13.

24. Materson BJ et al for the Department of Veterans Affairs Cooperative Study Group on Antihypertensive Agents. Single-drug therapy for hypertension in men. A comparison of six antihypertensive agents with placebo. N Engl J Med 1993; 328: 914–21.

25. Guidelines Committee. 2003 European Society of Hypertension – European Society of Cardiology guidelines for the management of arterial hypertension. J Hypertens 2003; 21: 1011–53.

26. Hansson L, Zanchetti S, Carruthers S, Dahlof B, Elmfeldt D, Julius S et al for the HOT Study Group. Effects of intensive blood pressure lowering and low-dose aspirin in patients with hypertension: principal results of the Hypertension Optimal Treatment (HOT) randomised trial. Lancet 1998; 351: 1755–62.

27. Tight blood pressure control and risk of macrovascular and microvascular complications in type 2 diabetes: UKPDS 38. Br Med J 1998; 317: 703–13.

28. Cappuccio FP, Markandu ND, Tucker FA, Shore AC, McGregor GA. A double blind study of the blood-pressure lowering effect of a thiazide diuretic in hypertensive patients already on nifedipine and a beta-blocker. J Hypertens 1987; 5: 733–8.

29. Primatesta P, Brookes M, Poulter NR. Improved hypertension management and control. Results from the Health Survey for England 1998. Hypertension 2001; 38: 827–32.

30. Brown MJ, Cruickshank JK, Dominiczak AF et al. Better blood pressure control: how to combine drugs. J Hum Hypertens 2003; 17: 81–6.

31. Williams B, Poulter N, Brown M et al. Guidelines for management of hypertension: report of the fourth working party of the British Hypertension Society, 2004 – BHS IV. 2004 (in press).

32. The JNC7 Report. The Seventh Report of the Joint National Committee on Prevention, Detection, Evaluation, and Treatment of High Blood Pressure. JAMA 2003; 289: 2560–72.

33. Parving H-H, Lehnert H, Brochner-Mortensen J, Gomis R, Andersen S, Arner P for the Irbesartan in Patients with Type 2 Diabetes and Microalbuminuria Study Group. The effect of irbesartan on the development of diabetic nephropathy in patients with type 2 diabetes. N Engl J Med 2001; 345: 870–8.

34. Brenner BM, Cooper ME, de Zeeuw D et al for the RENAAL Study Investigators. Effects of losartan on renal and cardiovascular outcomes in patients with type 2 diabetes and nephropathy. N Engl J Med 2001; 345: 861–9.

35. Lewis EJ, Hunsicker LG, Clarke WR et al for the Collaborative Study Group. Renoprotective effects of the angiotensin-receptor antagonists irbesartan in patients with nephropathy due to type 2 diabetes. N Engl J Med 2001; 345: 851–60.

36. Lindholm LH, Ibsen H, Dahlof B et al for the LIFE Study Group. Cardiovascular morbidity and mortality in patients with diabetes in the Losartan Intervention For Endpoint reduction in hypertension study (LIFE): a randomised trial against atenolol. Lancet 2002; 359: 1004–10.

37. Williams B. The renin-angiotensin system and cardiovascular disease: Hope or Hype? JRAAS 2000; 1: 142–6.

38. Dahlof B, Pennert K, Hansson L. Reversal of left ventricular hypertrophy in hypertensive patients: A meta-analysis of 109 treatment studies. Am J Hypertens 1992; 5: 95–110.

39. Jennings G, Wong J. Regression of left ventricular hypertrophy in hypertension: changing patterns with successive meta-analyses. J Hypertens 1998; 6(Suppl): S29–34.

40. The Heart Outcomes Prevention Evaluation Study Investigators. Effects of an angiotensin-converting-enzyme inhibitor, ramipril, on cardiovascular events in high-risk patients. N Engl J Med 2000; 342: 145–53.

41. Svenson P, de Faire U, Sleight P, Yusuf S, Ostergren J. Comparative effects of ramipril on ambulatory and office blood pressures; a HOPE Substudy. Hypertension 2001; 38: e28.

42. MacMahon S, Neal B, Tzouirion et al for the PROGRESS Collaborative Group. Randomised trial of a perindopril-based blood-pressure-lowering regimen among 6105 individuals with previous stroke or transient ischaemic attack. Lancet 2001; 358: 1033–41.

43. PATS Collaborative Group. Post-stroke antihypertensive treatment study. Clin Med J 1995; 108: 710–17.

Chapter 7

What concomitant therapy is needed?

Which patients with hypertension merit lipid-lowering therapy?

Two trials – the Antihypertensive and Lipid-Lowering Treatment to Prevent Heart Attack Trial (ALLHAT-LLT)[1] and the Anglo-Scandinavian Cardiac Outcomes Trial – Lipid Lowering Arm (ASCOT-LLA)[2] – have recently evaluated the benefits associated with the use of statins, specifically among patients with hypertension. Prior to these trial results, other randomised, controlled trial data were available from analyses of the hypertensive sub-groups in lipid-lowering trials in secondary and primary prevention and from the largest statin trial, the Heart Protection Study (HPS).[3] In the HPS, 41% of the patients were hypertensive, but 62% of the elderly patients in the Pravastatin in elderly individuals at risk of vascular disease (PROSPER) trial[4] were hypertensive. This trial, like HPS, mainly included patients with established vascular disease. Analyses of the hypertensive sub-groups from these trials demonstrate that the benefits of lipid lowering, primarily with statins, in terms of preventing major cardiovascular events are similar for hypertensive and normotensive patients (Table 7.1). Somewhat more surprising is the finding that in the statin trials stroke risk was reduced by an average of about 15% and 30% in primary and secondary prevention settings, respectively.[5]

Trial	1°/2°	Treated hypertension		Not hypertensive	
		n	End-point	n	End-point
4S*	2°	1154	-37%	4444	-34%
CARE*	2°	1774	-23%	4159	-24%
LIPID*	2°	3758	-15%	9014	-24%
GREACE*	2°	686	-48%	1600	-51%
HPS†	1°+2°	10594	-20%	20536	-24%
PROSPER†	1°+2°	2212	-15%	5804	-15%
WOSCOPS*	1°	1037	?	6595	-31%
AFCAPS/TexCAPS*	1°	1445	-39%	6605	-37%

End-point* CHD †CHD + stroke

Table 7.1 Randomised clinical trials of statins.

ALLHAT-LLT and ASCOT-LLA studies

ALLHAT-LLT compared the impact of 40 mg/day pravastatin with usual care in over 10,000 hypertensive patients (see Fig. 6.2) The differential effect of pravastatin on total – and LDL – cholesterol (11% and 17%, respectively) was smaller than expected due to extensive statin use in the usual care group and was associated with a modest, non-significant 9% reduction in fatal coronary heart disease (CHD) and non-fatal myocardial infarction (MI), and a 9% reduction in fatal and non-fatal stroke. No impact on all-cause mortality – the primary end-point of the trial – was apparent. By contrast, the results of ASCOT-LLA (Fig. 6.9), which also included over 10,000 hypertensive patients, showed highly significant cardiovascular benefits (36% reduction in the primary end-point of total CHD and non-fatal MI and a 27% reduction in fatal and non-fatal stroke) associated with the use of atorvastatin 10 mg/day compared with placebo in patients with total cholesterol ≤ 6.5 mmol/l. In addition, highly significant reductions in total cardiovascular events (21%) and total coronary events (29%) were observed. The difference in effects on cardiovascular outcomes seen in ALLHAT-LLT and ASCOT-LLA probably reflects the greater relative difference in total – and LDL – cholesterol (24% and 35%, respectively) achieved among the actively treated groups in ASCOT-LLA.

The HPS included only 1% of patients who were hypertensive but did not have either a history of a cardiovascular event, active vascular disease, and/or diabetes, and hence does not provide a robust database on which to base recommendations for primary prevention of cardiovascular disease (CVD) with lipid-lowering agents in hypertensive patients. However, in view of the results of ASCOT-LLA and other currently available trial data it seems reasonable to treat all those patients with hypertension at least up the age of 80 years with a total cholesterol > 3.5 mmol/l (135 mg/dl) who have established vascular disease or, in the context of primary prevention, an estimated 10-year cardiovascular risk of 20% (15% CHD) or more with a statin. Indeed these recommendations, along with more aggressive lipid targets (< 4 mmol/l total cholesterol or < 2 mmol/l LDL) have been incorporated into the recent ESH-ESC guidelines for hypertension management.[6]

Which patients with hypertension should receive aspirin?

The recommendations made in the 1999 British Hypertension Society (BHS) guidelines[7] regarding the use of aspirin appear to be a very reasonable interpretation of the best available data so far:

1. For *primary prevention*: 75 g aspirin/day is recommended for hypertensive patients aged 50 years or older who have controlled BP to at least < 150/90 mmHg and either target-organ damage or diabetes or a 10-year coronary heart disease risk of ≥ 15% (equivalent to a 10-year CVD risk of ≥ 20%).

2. For *secondary prevention:* (i.e. when there is established CVD, e.g. angina, MI, ischaemic stroke, TIA, or peripheral arterial disease): 75 mg of aspirin is recommended.

Which patients with hypertension should receive antioxidant therapy?

An important mechanistic role of antioxidants has been clearly identified in the development of atherosclerosis.[8] However to date, there are no trial data to support the use of any antioxidant for patients with hypertension unless they suffer from a nutritional deficiency.

The largest trial to date to evaluate the effects of vitamins on cardiovascular events was the Heart Protection Study (HPS),[9] which in a factorial design evaluated the impact of a combination of vitamins (vitamin E, vitamin C and beta-carotene) compared with placebo in over 20,000 patients at high risk of developing a cardiovascular event. Figure 7.1 confirms the lack of benefit of the antioxidant vitamins on any of the fatal end-points measured. Importantly over 8000 of the HPS trial population were hypertensive and in this large sub-group of HPS, vitamins were equally ineffective.

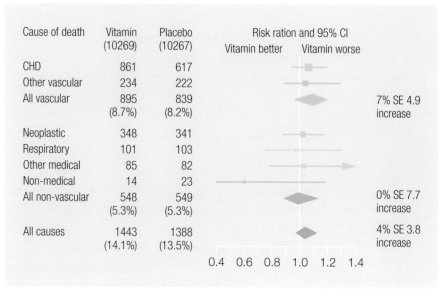

Figure 7.1 Vitamin: Cause-specific mortality in HPS.[9]

Summary

- Lipid lowering with statins should be provided to all those patients with hypertension and an estimated total 10 year CVD risk ≥20%.

- Asprin should be provided to all those with established CV disease (assuming no contraindications e.g. bleeding propensity etc).

- In the context of primary prevention asprin should be supplied only once specified conditions are satisfied (i.e. age >50 years, controlled BP and 10 year CVD ≥20%).

- Vitamin supplements are of no value except for treating a nutritional deficiency.

References

1. The ALLHAT Officers and Coordinators for the ALLHAT Collaborative Research Group. Major outcomes in moderately hypercholesterolemic, hypertensive patients randomized to pravastatin vs usual care. The Antihypertensive and Lipid-Lowering Treatment to Prevent Heart Attack Trial (ALLHAT-LLT). JAMA 2002; 288: 2998–3007.

2. Sever PS, Dahlof B, Poulter NR et al for the ASCOT investigators. Prevention of coronary and stroke events with atorvastatin in hypertensive patients who have average or lower-than-average cholesterol concentrations, in the Anglo-Scandinavian Cardiac Outcomes Trial – Lipid Lowering Arm (ASCOT-LLA): a multicentre randomised controlled trial. Lancet 2003; 361: 1149–58.

3. Heart Protection Study Group. MRC/BHF Heart Protection Study of cholesterol lowering with simvastatin in 20,536 high-risk individuals: a randomised placebo-controlled trial. Lancet 2002; 360: 7–22.

4. Shepherd J, Blauw GJ, Murphy MB et al. Pravastatin in elderly individuals at risk of vascular disease (PROSPER): a randomised controlled trial. Lancet 2002; 360: 1623–30.

5. Crouse JR, Byington RP, Furberg CD. HMG-CoA reductase inhibitor therapy and stroke risk reduction: an analysis of clinical trials data. Atherosclerosis 1998; 138: 11–24.

6. Guidelines Committee. 2003 European Society of Hypertension – European Society of Cardiology guidelines for the management of arterial hypertension. J Hypertens 2003; 21: 1011–53.

7. Ramsay LE, Williams B, Johnston GD et al. Guidelines for Management of Hypertension: Report of the third working party of the British Hypertension Society, 1999. J Human Hypertens 1999; 13: 569–92.

8. Diaz MZ, Frei B, Vita JA, Keaney JF Jr. Antioxidants and atherosclerotic heart disease. N Engl J Med 1997; 337: 408–16.

9. Heart Protection Study Collaborative Group. MRC/BHF Heart Protection Study of cholesterol lowering with simvastatin in 20,536 high-risk individuals: a randomised placebo-controlled trial. Lancet 2002; 360:7-22.

Chapter 8

How to improve BP control

How well is BP treated and controlled?

Contemporary surveys from all over the world[1-3] are consistent in showing that BP control (as defined by being below currently recommended targets) is achieved only in a small minority of patients with levels of BP currently considered as hypertensive. Table 8.1 shows rates of awareness, treatment and control from four countries around the world.[4]

Why is hypertension managed so inadequately?

Possible explanations for the levels of control shown in Table 8.1 are shown in Table 8.2.

Each of these possible explanations for poor BP control is likely to contribute to a variable degree. Rates of compliance or adherence

		Hypertension awareness in the population (%)	Hypertension treatment in the population (%)	Hypertension control in the population (%)	Hypertension control in treated hypertensives (%)
USA	Total	69.3	52.5	28.6	54.5
	Men	62.5	43.5	19.9	45.8
	Women	77.0	62.5	38.3	61.2
Canada	Total	63.2	36.4	17.2	47.3
	Men	57.0	27.6	9.8	35.6
	Women	69.4	45.1	24.5	54.3
England	Total	35.8	24.8	10.0	40.3
	Men	34.1	23.2	9.2	39.7
	Women	37.5	26.4	10.7	40.5
Germany	Total	36.5	26.1	7.8	29.9
	Men	32.5	22.6	5.8	25.7
	Women	?	?	?	?

Table 8.1 Age-adjusted hypertension awareness, treatment and control in the population, and control in treated hypertensive patients in %, 35–64 years, at the 160/90 mmHg threshold.[4]

and persistence with therapy have been reported in several settings and been shown to be low. Non-randomised observational follow-up data suggest that after initiation of monotherapy with each of the standard agents, only a minority are still taking the therapy after 1 year. This lack of persistence can be explained by several reasons, including lack of drug efficacy, side effects, drug costs and presumably a perception by the patient and/or doctor that continued treatment is not important. Some or all of these reasons may apply. Regarding BP-lowering efficacy and side effects, there is no doubt that individuals respond differently to different drug classes, and it is true that in a very small proportion of patients BP is resistant to therapy. In different health care settings the cost of drugs is not acceptable to the patient and hence the patient may feel that any marginal benefits of treatment are not worth the cost. Similarly it is easier and cheaper, at least short term, for the prescribing doctor not to bother to ensure careful follow up of patients and the BP treatment.

Paradoxically the production of guidelines on hypertension management can produce an adverse impact on BP management. This comes about because among the plethora of guidelines produced, there are potentially several on hypertension (e.g. WHO-ISH,[5] BHS,[6] JNC 7[7], ESH-ESC[8]) that might reach the general practitioner or hospital practitioner. These guidelines have historically differed from each other, which causes confusion and frustration, and which in turn may lead to inertia. However,

- Poor compliance
- Drug side-effects
- Ineffective drugs
- Physician inertia
- Drug costs
- Guideline confusion
- Resistant hypertension

Table 8.2 Reasons for inadequate control of BP.

even if the guidelines were consistent in all critical aspects, they all suffer from a common feature – length and complexity. This guarantees that they are not read and/or followed.

Whilst all the excuses shown in Table 8.2 do apply to one extent or another, the net result is invariably inadequate control with an associated intolerable burden of excess cardiovascular events. Among these excuses, perhaps the most important and remediable target for improving the status quo regarding BP levels, is that of physician inertia. For example, it has been established that, despite evidence of the need for at least two agents to achieve BP control (Chapter 6, p. 78), 60% of patients currently on treatment for raised BP in England are on one drug.[1] Further, a large European survey showed that, when faced with patients not at BP targets (as determined by the physician) 84% of such patients receive a repeat prescription (Fig. 8.2).

In short, the reasons for poor BP control may be valid to one extent or another, and clearly several of these reasons are interrelated. Nevertheless, most of these problems can be minimised by good clinical practice, as outlined in any of the major sets of guidelines.

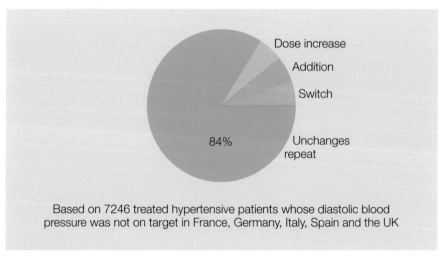

Based on 7246 treated hypertensive patients whose diastolic blood pressure was not on target in France, Germany, Italy, Spain and the UK

Figure 8.2 Treatment strategy adopted in hypertensive patients in whom target blood pressure is not achieved.

Can we improve BP control?

In short, the answer to this question, as intimated above, is an unequivocal yes.

One fundamental approach, and ultimately the most appealing and appropriate way of improving BP control, is to pre-empt the development of raised BP. This is dependent upon a population strategy designed to shift the mean BP of the population downwards. If the mean BP of the population is reduced, the proportion of hypertensive patients will be reduced as shown by the data in Figure 8.3. These data from the Intersalt study show that the mean of the population variable predicts the proportion of the extreme of that variable. Only a small shift in mean population BP (e.g. 3 mmHg) is required to generate a bigger benefit in terms of cardiovascular events saved, compared with the high-risk policy currently recommended (i.e. finding and treating those with a BP over a given threshold). It seems likely that non-drug manoeuvres can produce such a sufficiently large BP reduction if they were generally implemented (see Ch. 4, p. 53).

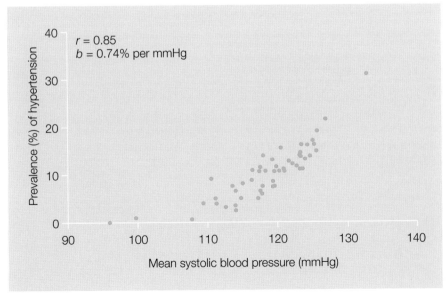

Figure 8.3 Relationship between population mean systolic BP and the prevalence of hypertension across 52 population samples from 32 countries.

For such an effect to be achieved however, major interventions by governments in association with schools, the food industry, and through legislation are required. Meanwhile the action necessary by and in the direct remit of practicing physicians are outlined in Table 8.2.

1	Improve screening of BP (see Ch. 2, p. 106)
2	Provide and reinforce effective, individually sensitive and targeted non-pharmacological advice (see Ch. 4, p. 54)
3	Explain why effective BP management and control is important for the patient
4	Establish whether the patient wishes to reduce the adverse effects of raised BP.
5	Initiate drug treatment if BP thresholds are exceeded despite non-drug measures (see Ch. 3, p. 45 and Ch. 6, p. 66)
6	Warn patients that two or more drugs are likely to be needed and that if side effects occur alternative drugs can be used
7	Continue to supply and enforce non-drug advice
8	Ask carefully about side effects
9	Titrate and modify drug regimens on the basis of BP-lowering efficacy (see Ch. 6, p. 76) but adjust as required if side effects occur
10	Titrate drugs as required to reach BP targets (see Ch. 5, p. 62)
11	Follow-up patients regularly until control is achieved. Once BP is controlled, follow-up should be on a regular basis (three to four times/ year) with repeat BP measures, preferably carried out by a nurse under standardised conditions (after 5 minutes' rest, sitting, correct cuff etc.)

Table 8.2 How to improve BP control.

Summary

- BP treatment in the developed world currently suboptimal and worse in the developing world.

- Most patients require at least two antihypertensive agents to reach current targets. Patients and their physicians should acknowledge this.

- Non drug treatment should be recommended and implemented to reduce the number or doses of drugs used.

References

1. Primatesta P, Brookes M, Poulter NR. Improved hypertension management and control. Results from the Health Survey for England 1998. Hypertension 2001; 38: 827–32.

2. Burt VL, Whelton P, Roccella EL et al. Prevalence of hypertension in the US adult population: results from the Third National Health and Nutrition Examination Survey, 1988–1991. Hypertension 1995; 25: 305–13.

3. Kastarinen MU, Salomaa VV, Vartiainen EA et al. Trends in blood pressure levels and control of hypertension in Finland from 1982–1997. J Hypertens 1998; 16: 1379–87.

4. Wolf-Maier K, Cooper RS, Kramer H, Banegas JR, Giampaoli S, Joffres MR, Poulter N, Primatesta P, Stegmayr B, Thamm M. Hypertension treatment and control in five European countries, Canada, and the United States. Hypertension 2004;43:10-17.

5. WHO-ISH Writing Group. 2003 WHO/ISH statement on management of hypertension (in press).

6. Bryan Williams, Neil R Poulter, Morris J Brown, Mark Davis, Gordon T McInnes, John F Potter, Peter S Sever, and Simon McG Thom. British Hypertension Society guidelines for hypertension management 2004 (BHS-IV): summary. BMJ 2004;328:634-640.

7. The JNC7 Report. The Seventh Report of the Joint National Committee on Prevention, Detection, Evaluation, and Treatment of High Blood Pressure. JAMA 2003; 289: 2560–72.

8. Guidelines Committee. 2003 European Society of Hypertension – European Society of Cardiology guidelines for the management of arterial hypertension. J Hypertens 2003; 21: 1011–53.

Chapter 9

What are the prospects for the future?

What don't we know?

Despite having the results of almost 30 major morbidity and mortality trials,[1] many of which have been published since 1993, the answers to most of the outstanding questions which prevailed in 1993 remain unanswered (see Ch. 6, p. 65).

Confusion remains as to optimal first-line therapy (see Ch. 6, p. 67) and whilst it seems reasonable to recommend low-dose diuretics as a starting point for many patients, the trial evidence for using low-dose thiazides in this context is by no means compelling except for cost reasons. Furthermore it is inherently unlikely, given the heterogeneity of the hypertensive population, that any one drug is the best for all sub-groups and types of patient. However, given the need in most patients for at least two agents to control blood pressure (BP) effectively, more trials of pairs of antihypertensive agents are required, and ideally they are required in the setting of different patient sub-groups (e.g. those with LVH, diabetes etc.).

It seems unlikely that validation of treating low-risk patients with a systolic BP in the range of 140–159 in a placebo-controlled trial will be carried out. However the randomised trial evidence for so doing is not available and the cost implications of this policy (already effectively a worldwide recommendation) is massive. The trade-off of risk and benefit in this group should be evaluated in a trial.

The shortcomings of the Hypertension Optimal Treatment (HOT) trial[2] were outlined in Chapter 5 and highlight the need for a more definitive trial focused on systolic targets given the greater predictive value of systolic BP for most patients wih hypertension. The need for such a trial was included in the WHO-ISH guidelines produced in 1999,[3] which outlined the need for further research in eight areas (Table 9.1). Most of these areas are being addressed in the many ongoing trials.[5] However, perhaps the most important glaring omission is work in the developing world. As described in Chapter 1, p. 6, this is the critical target for preventing the anticipated increase in the burden of hypertension and cardiovascular diseases in the next 2 decades. The potential for primordial prevention and improved BP management remains but only if suitable research is designed, resourced, and carried out urgently.

- BP and CVD in developing countries
- Alternative BP measurement
- BP lowering in high-risk patients
- More versus less BP lowering
- Evaluation of surrage end-points
- Combined interventions for CVD prevention
- Effects of newer BP lowering agents
- Genetically targeted BP lowering therapy

Table 9.1 1999 WHO–ISH guidelines: Recommended areas for future research.

In the most recent hypertension guidelines (except JNC 7)[4] thresholds for treating hypertension are increasingly based on estimated cardiovascular risk. It should be acknowledged however that no trials have been designed to include patients on the basis of a specific level of risk. Hence it is difficult and perhaps inappropriate, pending such information, to replace BP levels by risk levels when making treatment recommendations.

How to improve implementation of guidelines

Suggestions for improving BP control at the individual level are outlined in Chapter 8, p. 103 (Table 8.2). However at a population level the advice given to the general public and those responsible for healthcare delivery needs to improve dramatically. Public education on health is achievable. Despite some cynical views regarding large population-based interventions, startling beneficial effects on cardiovascular disease (CVD) and mortality have been demonstrated at the population level. For example in Finland, the reduction in cardiovascular deaths over a 20-year period, following a broad-based national campaign to improve diet and lifestyles (Fig. 9.1) appears to have been almost completely attributable to the healthy life changes that were made.[6]

The improved implementation of guidelines necessitates more effective communication between those producing the guidelines and the healthcare professionals charged with managing patients. It may also be useful to produce documents, written, visual, or electronic, designed to inform the general public. Key features of ideal guidelines are shown in Table 9.2. In the interests of optimal broad-based uptake of guidelines, a pivotal component required is simplicity. Brief, simple messages with the

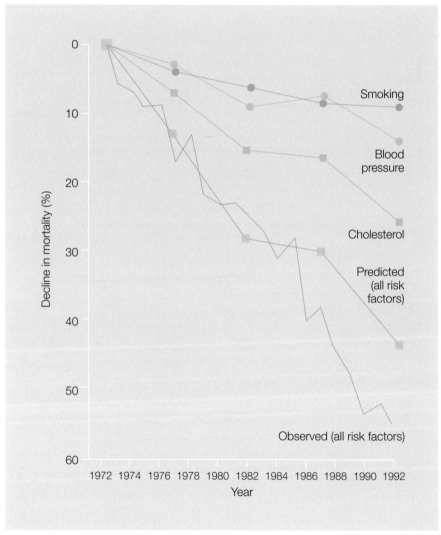

Figure 9.1 Observed and predicted decline in mortality from ischemic heart disease in men aged 35–64 in Finland.[6]

inevitable trade-off of a degree of inaccuracy are required. For example it has been suggested that drug intervention be based on a systolic BP level of 150 mmHg.[7] Levels above this should be treated and the target should be below 150 mmHg. Not much is lost by ignoring diastolic BP except among the young, and whilst perhaps conservative, achieving this level of 'control' in the vast majority of those with hypertension would constitute a major improvement in BP management in countries such as the UK.[8] In the context of developing countries with restricted resources, such a policy may well have major advantages over trying to implement more aggressive guidelines produced out of context.

Will more effective modification become available?

There is a continuing need for more effective agents from among currently available drug classes, ideally with fewer side effects. Perhaps more importantly newer classes of agents are required and several new classes of agents are being developed. To provide real advances over currently available agents, such products will be required to have long duration of action and low side-effect rates, with BP-lowering efficacy associated with commensurate reduction in cardiovascular events. The benefits of pharmacogenetics whereby drugs may be targeted on the basis of genetic profiling are considered by some to be on the horizon, others

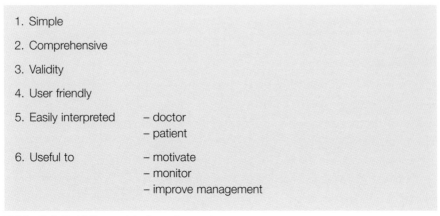

1. Simple

2. Comprehensive

3. Validity

4. User friendly

5. Easily interpreted   – doctor
                                    – patient

6. Useful to   – motivate
                                    – monitor
                                    – improve management

Table 9.2 Guidelines – ideal requirements.

believe this is a rather distant horizon. Meanwhile with the increasing need and use of polypharmacy in an ageing population, the trends are likely to move further towards the use of combination therapies. This is likely to involve not just combination of two (or more) antihypertensive agents as discussed in Chapter 6, p. 78 but also the combination of various products which act on different cardiovascular risk factors.

The need for such products is highlighted by the typical drug requirements of a diabetic patient who has suffered a myocardial infarction. The minimum drug requirements for such a patient include aspirin, statin, one (or more) oral hypoglycaemic agent, a beta-blocker, an angiotensin-converting enzyme (ACE) inhibitor, and a fish oil preparation. This patient may also need further BP-lowering agents, a fibrate, and insulin.

Clearly compliance would be enhanced by combining some of these products into one tablet. Although by no means a new idea, this concept has been highlighted recently by publication of an article proposing the production of a 'polypill', which includes several different drug types.[9] In the context of high-risk patients, e.g. those with raised BP, a logical combination might include one or more effective BP lowering agents, a lipid-lowering agent and low-dose aspirin. However the requirements of a polypill for use in a population strategy – that is to give to everyone above a certain age – are more stringent. In short, the components should have a side-effect profile that is as close to that of a placebo as possible, since the risk–benefit ratio becomes less favourable at the population level. The benefits of each of the components must have been established in large randomised trials but large reductions in each of the risk factors to be targeted are not required (see Ch. 1, p. 16).

Of currently available products, the combination of an angiotensin II receptor blocker (ARB), a statin and possibly very low-dose aspirin, would best suit the requirements of a polypill for use in the whole population. However the polypill recently proposed[9] does not fit the ideal profile of such an agent since of the six agents to be combined, it includes folate (unproven to produce cardiovascular benefits in any trials as yet), beta-blockers, ACE inhibitors and diuretics (associated with frequent side effects including weight gain, small adverse lipid and glucose effects, wheezing in those with obstructive airways disease, cough, impotence, and urinary frequency). Furthermore the use of three antihypertensive agents would undoubtedly produce an unnecessarily large drop in BP in a proportion of "normaltensive" recipients with an associated significant incidence of hypotensive episodes. In the context of a population strategy, this combination may cause at least as much harm as good. In short, the most recently proposed polypill has major shortcomings for use in the whole population, whilst variations on a theme have real potential benefits for use in the high-risk context. Several combination products are in development or production and it seems likely that their availability will be greeted with enthusiasm by the increasing numbers who need to take several medications daily, and by those who prescribe them.

Population vs high-risk strategy

In conclusion, the data shown in Figure 9.2 are a startling reminder that the vast majority of adults aged 65 years and older have levels of BP which currently 'merit' BP-lowering treatment according to current guidance. Whilst there is a real need for more effective drug therapies to improve the control of risk factors such as raised BP or cholesterol, it cannot be right to accept as inevitable the age-related increase in risk factors and the mass medication and vast burden of disease which cardiovascular disease currently imposes. Only a population strategy to change diets and lifestyle from childhood onwards can avert the current situation and the anticipated global expansion of this problem.

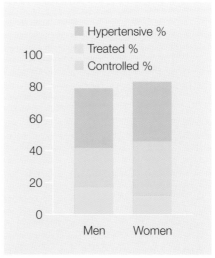

Figure 9.2 HSE 2000 – elderly hypertensive*, treated and controlled (* i.e. ≥140/90 mmHg).

Meanwhile physicians are duty-bound to at least inform the patients of benefits likely to arise from the prudent and appropriate use of currently available agents shown in randomised trials to greatly reduce the risk of cardiovascular events.

Summary

■ BP levels and hence hypertension prevalence will worsen over the next two decades.

■ Trials to fill some outstanding gaps in our knowledge are still required.

■ More effective guideline implementation is required.

■ A population strategy is sorely needed to reduce the burden of hypertension.

■ Increase use of combinations of therapies can be anticipated.

References

1. Blood Pressure Lowering Treatment Trialists' Collaboration. Effects of different blood-pressure-lowering regimens on major cardiovascular events: results of prospectively-designed overviews of randomised trials. Lancet 2003;362:1527-35.

2. Hansson L, Zanchetti S, Carruthers S et al for the HOT Study Group. Effects of intensive blood pressure lowering and low-dose aspirin in patients with hypertension: principal results of the Hypertension Optimal Treatment (HOT) randomised trial. Lancet 1998; 351: 1755–62.

3. Guidelines Subcommittee. 1999 World Health Organization– International Society of Hypertension Guidelines for the Management of Hypertension. J Hypertens 1999; 17: 151–83.

4. The JNC7 Report. The Seventh Report of the Joint National Committee on Prevention, Detection, Evaluation, and Treatment of High Blood Pressure. JAMA 2003; 289: 2560–72.

5. World Health Organization – International Society of Hypertension Blood Pressure Lowering Treatment Trialists' Collaboration. Protocol for prospective collaborative overviews of major randomized trials of blood-pressure-lowering treatments. J Hypertens 1998; 16: 127.

6. Vartiainen E, Puska P, Pekkanen J, Tuomilehto J, Jousilahti P. Changes in risk factors explain changes in mortality from ischaemic heart disease in Finland. Br Med J 1994; 309: 23–7.

7. Sever P. Simple blood pressure guidelines for primary health care. J Human Hypertens 1999; 13: 725–7.

8. Primatesta P, Brookes M, Poulter NR. Improved hypertension management and control. Results from the Health Survey for England 1998. Hypertension 2001; 38: 827–32.

9. Wald NJ, Law MR. A strategy to reduce cardiovascular disease by more than 80%. Br Med J 2003; 326: 1419–24.

Index

Indexer: Dr Laurence Errington

Abbreviations used:
BP, blood pressure
CV, cardiovascular

A

ABCD approach (drug combinations),
80-2
ABCD trials, 61
ACE inhibitors *see* angiotensin-
converting enzyme inhibitors
adherence *see* compliance
Adult Treatment Panel III *see* National
Cholesterol Education Program/
Adult Treatment Panel III
aetiology (cause) and risk factors, 9-13
secondary hypertension *see* secondary
hypertension
AFCAPS/TexCAPS, 96
African descent, persons of, aetiology
in, 11
age distribution, 5-9
Air Force/Texas Coronary
Atherosclerosis Prevention Study
(AFCAPS/TexCAPS), 96
aldosterone antagonist, ALLHAT study,
77
ALLHAT *see* Antihypertensive Therapy
and Lipid Lowering Heart Attack
Prevention Trial
alpha-blockers
ALLHAT study, 62, 70, 71, 72, 77, 80
beta-blockers combined with, 80
ambulatory BP measurement, 26, 28
amlodipine
ALLHAT study, 70, 73
IDNT study, 86
ANBP2, 74-5
angiotensin-converting enzyme (ACE)
inhibitors
ALLHAT study, 62, 70, 71-2, 72, 73,
77
ANBP2 study, 74
Blood Pressure Lowering Treatment
Trialists Collaboration, 75

CAPPP study, 68-9
combined with other drugs, 81-2, 82,
114
diabetic, post-myocardial infarction,
114
HOPE study, 88
PROGRESS study, 88-9
salt restriction combined with, 56
STOP-2 study, 69
UKPDS study, 85
see also specific agents
angiotensin II receptor blockers
(ARBs), 76, 85-6, 87-8
ALLHAT study, 77
combined with other drugs, 114
in diabetes/diabetic nephropathy, 45,
85-6
salt restriction combined with, 56
Anglo-Scandinavian Cardiac Outcome
Trial (ASCOT), 75, 82
design, 84
lipid-lowering arm (LLA), 96, 97
antihypertensive drugs, 43-52, 59-94
combinations, 114-15
optimal, 67, 78-82
contemporary vs standard agents, 67,
67-78
costs, 78
failure, reasons, 102-4
first-line choice, 76-8, 110
future prospects, 109-17
initiating use, guidance, 44-52
variations, 48-9
mass use in elderly, 49
non-drug measures combined with,
56
in sub-groups of patients, 67, 83-8
target BP levels, 59-64
Antihypertensive Therapy and Lipid
Lowering Heart Attack Prevention
Trial (ALLHAT), 62, 70-4, 74, 80,
96, 97
diabetics, 85
lipid-lowering drugs in, 70, 96, 97
summary of, 77
antioxidants, 98

Appropriate Blood Pressure Control in
    Diabetes (ABCD) trials, 61
arrhythmias, ventricular, 18
ASCOT *see* Anglo-Scandinavian Cardiac
    Outcome Trial
aspirin, 98, 114
assessment, patient, 25-42
atenolol
    LIFE trial, 87
    UKPDS trial, 85
atorvastatin (in Greek Atorvastatin and
    Coronary-heart-disease Evaluation
    study), 96
Australian National BP Study-2, 74-5

B

beta-blockers
    ALLHAT study, 77
    combined with other drugs, 81, 82,
        114
    alpha-blockers, 80
    diabetic, post-myocardial infarction,
        114
    LIFE study, 87
    NORDIL study, 70
    STOP-2 study, 69
    UKPDS study, 85
black African populations, aetiology, 11
blood pressure
    control, 102
        future prospects, 109-17
        improving, 105-6
    CV disease risk prediction, 13-14, 20-1
    levels defining hypertension, 2-5
    mean
        geographical distribution, 7-9
        shifting downwards, 105
    measurement, 26-9
    target levels, 59-64
    see also diastolic BP; systolic BP
Blood Pressure Lowering Treatment
    Trialists (BPLT) Collaboration, 75
British Hypertension Society (BHS)
    risk assessment charts, 38
    tests recommended, 32

treatment guidelines, 45, 48
    BP targets, 62
    drug combinations, 80-2, 82

C

caffeine, 12
calcium channel blockers (CCBs), 68,
    76
    ALLHAT study, 70, 72, 73, 77
    dihydropyridine *see* dihydropyridine
    diuretics combined with, 79-80
    INSIGHT, 69
    NORDIL study, 70
    STOP-2 study, 69
    SYST-EUR study, 67-8
calcium intake, 12
Canada, awareness/treatment/control
    of hypertension in, 102
    see also United States and North
        America
CAPPP study, 68-9
captopril
    in CAPPP study, 68-9
    in UKPDS trial, 85
cardiac problems *see* heart
cardiovascular disease
    death, prediction, 35-6
    risk *see* risk
CARE study, 96
cause *see* aetiology
chlorthalidone, ALLHAT trial, 70, 72-4
cholesterol
    drugs lowering *see* lipid-lowering
        drugs
    raised, and raised BP, CV disease risk,
        20, 21-2
    fatal, SCORE project chart, 37
    see also HDL cholesterol; National
        Cholesterol Education Program
Cholesterol and Recurrent Events
    (CARE) study, 96
clinical trials *see* trials
cognitive impairment, 18-20
compliance (adherence), 114
    problems, 103-4

complications (disease; target organ damage) due to hypertension, 14-22
  signs of, 30, 31
coronary/ischaemic heart disease (and BP), 16-17
death/mortality
  cholesterol levels and, 21-2
  Finland, reduction, 112
  prediction, 35
  rates, 3, 15, 16
  risk prediction, 33, 34, 35, 36
  target BP levels in, 60
costs, antihypertensives, 78
cuff sizes, 27

D

death (mortality)
  coronary heart disease *see* coronary heart disease
  CV (in general)
    Finland, reduction, 111, 112
    prediction, 35-6
  sudden, hypertension and left ventricular hypertrophy and risk of, 18, 19
death rates
  coronary heart disease, and BP, 3, 15, 16
  in Multiple Risk Factor Intervention Trial, 14
  stroke, and BP, 3, 16
definition of hypertension, 2-5
dementia, 20
developmental stage (world), 9
diabetes, 83-6
  choice of antihypertensives, 83-5
  left ventricular hypertrophy and, 18
  MI patients with, drug requirements, 114
  renal disease/nephropathy, 17, 85-6
    angiotensin II receptor blockers, 45, 85-6
  risk assessment in, 33, 36
  target BP levels, 61

type 2/II, 84, 85-6
  diet and lifestyle interventions, 55
  in younger persons, rising incidence, 9
  in USA, epidemiology, 10
diastolic BP
  in CV disease prediction, 14
  in definition of hypertension, 4
  distribution, 6, 7
diet
  Finland, reducing CV deaths, 111
  as risk factor, 12
  therapeutic modifications, 54
dihydropyridine calcium channel blockers
  ALLHAT study, 70, 72, 73, 77
  combined with other drugs, 81
  INSIGHT study, 69
  SYST-EUR study, 67
diltiazem
  ALLHAT study, 77
  NORDIL study, 70
disease due to hypertension *see* complications
distribution of hypertension, 5-9
diuretics, 110
  ALLHAT study, 62, 70, 72-4, 77
  ANBP2 study, 74
  combined with other drugs, 81, 82, 114-15
    calcium channel blockers, 79-80
  LIFE study, 87
  NORDIL study, 70
  PROGRESS study, 88-9
  STOP-2 study, 69
domiciliary (home) BP measurement, 28-9
dose titration, antihypertensives, 78
doxazosin, 82
  ALLHAT study, 70, 71, 72
drug therapy
  antihypertensive *see* antihypertensive drugs
  compliance *see* compliance
  concomitant (non-antihypertensive), 67, 95-9, 114

dyslipidaemia coexisting with
  hypertension, 21

E

economic cost, antihypertensives, 78
elderly (over 65s)
  antihypertensives
    mass treatment, 49
    MRC trial, 68
  statins, 96
enalapril, ANBP2 study, 74
England, awareness/treatment/control
  of hypertension in, 102
  see also United Kingdom
environmental factors, 12, 13
  genetic factors interacting with, 9-10, 11
epidemiology, 1-24, 105
EUROPA trial, 62
Europe
  on coronary heart disease risk
    guidelines, 34
  means BPs, 7, 8
  treatment guidelines, 45, 47, 48-9
    drug combinations, 79-80, 82
European Society of Cardiology see
  European Society of Hypertension
  and European Society of
  Cardiology
European Society of Hypertension
  (ESH)
  BP measurement guidelines, 26-7
  definitions and classification of BP
    levels, 4, 5
European Society of Hypertension
  (ESH) and European Society of
  Cardiology (ESC)
  tests recommended by, 32
  treatment
    algorithms, 47
    BP targets, 62
    drug combinations, 79, 80
European trial On Reduction of
    cardiac events with Perindopril
    in Stable coronary Artery disease
    (EUROPA), 62

evaluation, patient, 25-42
examination, 30

F

females, prevalence in, 8
fibrates, 114
Finland, CV death reduction, 111, 112
folate, 114
4S trial (Scandinavian Simvastatin
    Survival Study), 96
Framingham study and coronary heart
  disease prediction, 34, 35

G

gender (sex) distribution, 5-9
genetic factors, 10-11
  environmental factors interacting, 9-
    10, 11
Germany, awareness/treatment/control
  of hypertension in, 102
global risk assessment, 31-8
GREACE (GREek Atorvastatin and
  Coronary-heart-disease Evaluation)
  study, 96
guidelines on hypertension
  management, 45-9
  adverse effects on BP management,
    103-4
  ideal requirements, 113
  improving implementation, 111-13
  on initiating use of antihypertensives
    see antihypertensive drugs
  see also specific guidelines

H

HDL cholesterol and coronary heart
  disease risk, 34, 35
heart disease, ischaemic see coronary
  heart disease
heart failure, 17
  BP lowering, 60
Heart Outcomes Prevention Evaluation
  (HOPE) study, 62, 88

Heart Protection Study, 96, 97, 98
high-density lipoprotein cholesterol and
    coronary heart disease risk, 34, 35
history-taking, 29, 30
home BP measurement, 28-9
HOPE study, 62, 88
HOT study, 61, 62, 78, 84, 110
HPS trial, 96, 97, 98
hydrochlorothiazide
    ANBP2 study, 74
    LIFE trial, 87
Hypertension Optimal Treatment
    (HOT) study, 61, 62, 78, 84, 110

I

IDNT study, 86-7
indapamide, PROGRESS trial, 88-9
insulin resistance syndrome, 9, 10
International Nifedipine GITS
    Study: Intervention as a Goal for
    Hypertension Treatment, 69-70
International Society of Hypertension-
    -WHO see World Health
    Organization
investigations, 30, 32
irbesartan
    IDNT study, 85-6
    IRMA2 study, 85
IRMA2, 85
ischaemic heart disease see coronary/
    ischaemic heart disease
isolated systolic hypertension, drug
    trial, 67-8

J

Joint British Recommendations, CV risk
    assessment, 38
    coronary heart disease, 34
Joint National Committee (JNC) on
    Prevention, Detection, Evaluation
    and Treatment of High BP
    definitions and classification of BP
        levels, 4, 5
    tests recommended by, 32

treatment
    algorithms, 46
    BP targets, 62
    drug combinations, 82
    risk classification in guidance for,
        31-3

K

kidney see renal disease

L

left ventricular hypertrophy, 17-18, 87
    antihypertensive choice, 87
    target BP levels, 60
LIFE study, 86, 87-8
lifestyle modification see non-
    pharmacological methods
lipid abnormalities coexisting with
    hypertension, 21
lipid-lowering drugs, 96-7
    ALLHAT study, 70, 96, 97
LIPID study, 96
lisinopril, ALLHAT study, 70, 73
Long-Term Intervention with
    Pravastatin in Ischaemic Disease
    (LIPID) study, 96
loop diuretics, ALLHAT study, 77
losartan trial, 86

M

macrovascular complications, 14
males, prevalence in, 8
medical history-taking, 29, 30
Medical Research Council (MRC),
    elderly, 68
men, prevalence in, 8
mercury sphygmomanometer, 27
meta-analyses, antihypertensives, 75-6
metabolic (insulin resistance)
    syndrome, 9, 10
mortality and mortality rates see death;
    death rates
MRC trial, elderly, 68

Multiple Risk Factor Intervention Trial, 14
myocardial infarction
  in diabetic, drug requirements, 114
  prevention in ALLHAT study, 70, 71
  risk
    hypertension and left ventricular hypertrophy and, 18, 19
    prediction, 35

N

National Cholesterol Education Program/Adult Treatment Panel III (NCEP/ATPIII) guidelines, 35
  diabetes and, 36
  metabolic syndrome defined, 9
natural history, 13-22
nephropathy see renal disease
nifedipine, INSIGHT study, 69
non-pharmacological methods (incl. lifestyle interventions), 12-13, 53-8
  drugs combined with, 56
  evidence for, 54-5
  Finland, reducing CV deaths, 111
Nordic Diltiazem Study (NORDIL), 70
North America see United States and North America

O

obesity
  epidemiology, 9, 10
  left ventricular hypertrophy and, 18
older people see elderly
organ damage, target see complications

P

palaeolithic diet, 13
perindopril trials
  EUROPA study, 62
  PROGRESS study, 62, 88-9
polypill, 114-15
population-based BP control strategies, 115

potassium intake, 12
pravastatin, 96, 97
  ALLHAT study, 70, 96, 97
prehypertension, definition, 4, 5
prevalence, 6-7, 105
PROGRESS, 62, 88-9
PROSPER trial, 97

R

ramipril, HOPE trial, 88
randomised controlled trials see trials
Reduction of Endpoints in NIDDM with the Angiotensin 2 Antagonist Losartan, 85-6
RENAAL, 85-6
renal disease (nephropathy), 17
  diabetes see diabetes
renin, 'high renin' vs 'low renin' hypertension, treatment recommendations, 81-2
risk (of CV disease)
  assessment/prediction, 31-8
  BP in, 14, 20-1
  global, 31-8
  drug therapy related to, 44-8, 66
  lifestyle interventions reducing, 55
risk factors for hypertension see aetiology

S

salt restriction, 56
Scandinavian Simvastatin Survival Study (4S), 96
SCORE project, 35-6, 37
secondary hypertension
  causes, 9-13
    identifying, 30
  forms and associations of, 12
sex distribution, 5-9
SHEP trial, 60, 67-8
simvastatin (in 4S trial - Scandinavian Simvastatin Survival Study), 964
smoking (and CV disease risk), 33
  raised BP and, 20, 21

reduction/cessation, 55
SCORE project chart, risk of fatality, 37
socioeconomic status, 7
sphygmomanometer, mercury, 27
statin, 96, 97
ALLHAT study, 70, 96, 97
combined with other drugs, 114
STOP-2, 69
stroke (BP and), 16-17
death/mortality
prediction, 35
rates, 3, 16
primary prevention trials, 96
risk prediction, 33, 34
secondary prevention trials, 88-9, 96
target BP levels following, 60
Swedish Trial in Older Patients with Hypertension-2, 69
SYST-EUR trial, 67-8
Systematic Coronary Risk Evaluation (SCORE) project, 35-6, 37
systolic BP
CV disease prediction and, 14
fatal, SCORE project chart, 37
in definition of hypertension, 4
distribution, 5, 6, 6-7
Europe vs N. America, 8
shifting the mean downwards, 105
Systolic hypertension, isolated, drug trial, 67-8
Systolic Hypertension in Europe Trial, 67-8
Systolic Hypertension in the Elderly Program (SHEP trial), 60, 67-8

T

tests and investigations, 30, 32
thiazide diuretics, 72-4, 110
ALLHAT study, 77
ANBP2 study, 74
STOP-2 study, 69
treatment, 12-13, 43-117
future prospects, 109-17
inadequacy, 102-4

JNC VI risk classification in guidance for, 31-3
non-pharmacological see non-pharmacological methods
pharmacological see drug therapy
target levels, 59-64
trials see trials
trials (incl. randomised controlled trials)
antihypertensives, 66-88
evidence as of 1993/94, 66-7
target BP levels, 60-2
antioxidants, 98
lipid-lowering drugs, 96, 97
24-hour (ambulatory) BP measurement, 26, 28

U

United Kingdom (UK)
treatment algorithms, 45, 48
UK Prospective Diabetes Study, 36, 61, 83-5
see also England
United States (USA) and North America
awareness/treatment/control of hypertension in, 102
diabetes and obesity trends, 10, 11
diet in, 13
means BPs, 7-9

V

vegetarian diet, 12
ventricular arrhythmias, 18
ventricular hypertrophy, left see left ventricular hypertrophy
verapamil, ALLHAT study, 77
vitamins, 98, 99

W

weight, body, 9
see also obesity
West of Scotland Coronary Prevention Study (WOSCOPS), 96

WHO *see* World Health Organization
women, prevalence in, 8
World Health Organization/
    International Society of
    Hypertension guidelines, 110, 111
    BP targets, 62
    risk stratification, 33
WOSCOPS (West of Scotland Coronary
    Prevention Study), 96